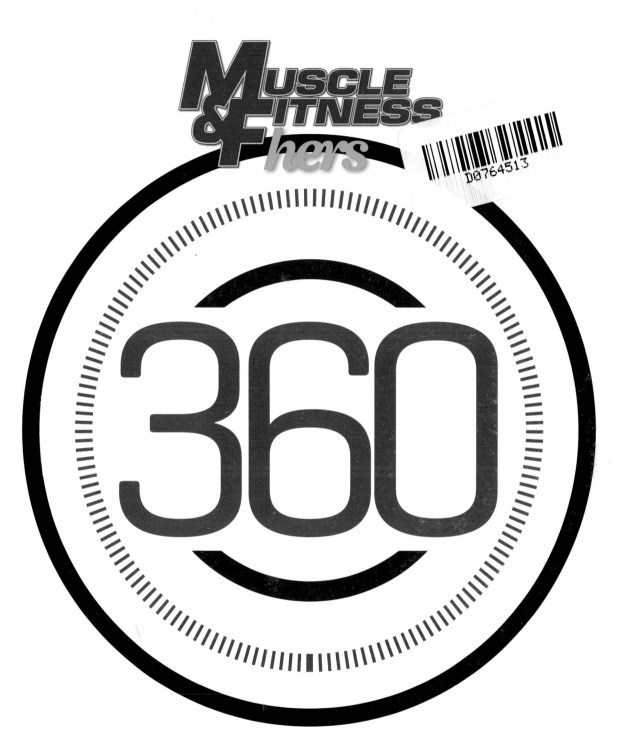

ACKNOWLEDGMENTS

This publication is based on articles written by **Rachel Cosgrove; Karla Dial; Mitzi Dulan; Jimmy Pena; Cat Perry; Sommer Roberston-Abiad; Carey Rossi; Amy Schlinger; Alyssa Shaffer; Jim Stoppani, Ph.D; Mark Thorpe; Eric Velazquez;** and **Joe Wuebben**

Cover photography by **Marc Royce**

Photography and illustrations by **Steve Boyle, Art Brewer, Tom Corbett, Michael Darter, Doron Gild, Ian Logan, Mike Medby, James Michelfelder, Jim Purdum, Marc Royce, Therese Sommerseth, Larissa Underwood,** and **Pavel Ythjall**

Project editor is **Joe Wuebben**

Project creative director is **Anthony Scerri**

Project copy editor is **Cat Perry**

Project photo assistant is **Anthony Nolan**

Founding chairman is **Joe Weider**. Chairman and CEO of American Media, Inc., is **David Pecker.**

This book is available in quantity at special discounts for your group or organization. For further information, contact:

Triumph Books
814 North Franklin Street
Chicago, IL 60610
(312) 337-0747
www.triumphbooks.com

ISBN: 978-1-60078-857-4

Printed in USA.

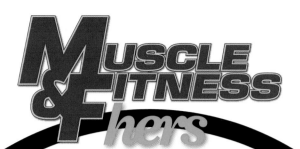

360

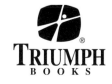

TRIUMPH
BOOKS

TRIUMPHBOOKS**.COM**

Contents

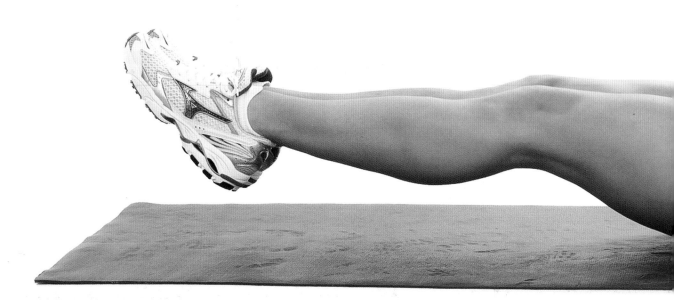

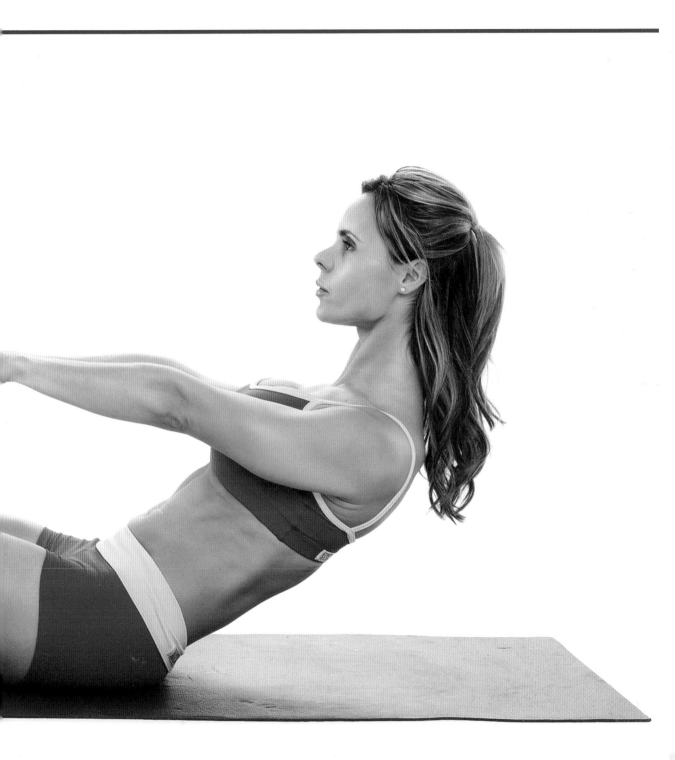

Foreword

THE FITNESS ADVANTAGE

Growing up in Romania, I never expected my life to flourish the way that it has. When I arrived in America as a teenager, I saw it as the gateway to opportunity. Attending school and working odd hours wasn't easy, but after years of hard work, I took on the monumental responsibilities of becoming a restaurant owner. But even while working long days and nights, I knew that I needed to make time for my health and fitness. That's when I stumbled upon a local gym. I began to train with a newfound intensity to balance the stress of my business, and, like all hardheaded Romanian women, I grew as competitive in the gym as I was in the restaurant business. At the urging of a trainer I entered my first figure competition.

I won that first show and eventually went on to earn my figure pro card. While most women don't need to take their commitment to fitness to a professional level, all of us need to make a pledge to embrace a healthy lifestyle. Looking and feeling your best means taking care of both body and mind, from eating right and moving more to finding the best way to cope with life's daily demands. When you treat yourself right, the rest all seems to fall into place.

This book is meant to serve as a 360-degree guide to helping you achieve these goals, whether it's through a regular workout routine; a clean, sensible diet; or smart ways to handle some of the daily stress and roadblocks that we all experience from time to time. For me, each day brings an opportunity to be healthy. I wake up early, grab a nutritious breakfast, and hit the gym. But it's not just my body that's getting stronger; the real success is harder to see. It's inside. Being active gives me confidence and informs how I approach daily problems, both small and large. Confidence makes you stand taller, with shoulders back and your face more relaxed. When you work hard to maintain your physical strength, your mental strength will never be far behind.

Confidence and mental and emotional resiliency are some of the key ingredients to a happier, more fulfilled life. And while happiness, of course, is often situational, it's also within your control, and it's cyclical. When you're happy, you exercise, and when you exercise, the results and positive feelings further encourage you to keep up with your routine. It's not always easy. At times, everyone has that "please just get me through this!" feeling, but try to remember the benefits. That sense of accomplishment and boost of energy will carry you through your day.

It is our goal that *Hers 360* can provide not just the tips and tools to help you get fit, but also the inspiration to become healthier and happier. You'll find fat-blasting training routines that will help you sculpt a strong, sexy body at home or at the gym. If you're looking to reshape a particular body part like your abs, arms, or glutes, *Muscle & Fitness Hers 360* will help you get there. And if time is a factor, this book provides super-speed express workouts that will help you get stronger and leaner in 30 minutes or less. For those who are looking to take their training to the next level, we've got proven intensity techniques guaranteed to deliver results. And there are diverse routines from other areas of fitness, including yoga and Olympic lifting.

Diet is a key component to achieving all of your better-body, better-health goals, so we've also put together the key information you need to keep you on track and make sure you can maximize your results without sabotaging your efforts.

I have my little indulgences at times, but too many in a row and I'm facing a downward spiral. I understand my personal formula by now: One bad meal is OK; two, and I tell myself I'll get back on the clean-eating wagon tomorrow. By the third slip, I'm disappointed and my mood dips by the hour. I know I'm not alone—everyone ebbs and flows between their good and bad habits. The good news is, it doesn't take much to get back on track; one day of clean eating and hard training is the beginning of a new you.

Besides the obvious advice of training hard and eating well, we also want to encourage you to walk with your head held high; remember to smile; and help someone in need, just because. I'm thrilled that you are willing to take this journey and hope that *Hers 360* will help you live a long, healthy, and happy life.

Yours in fitness,
MONA MURESAN
Editor-in-Chief
Muscle & Fitness Hers

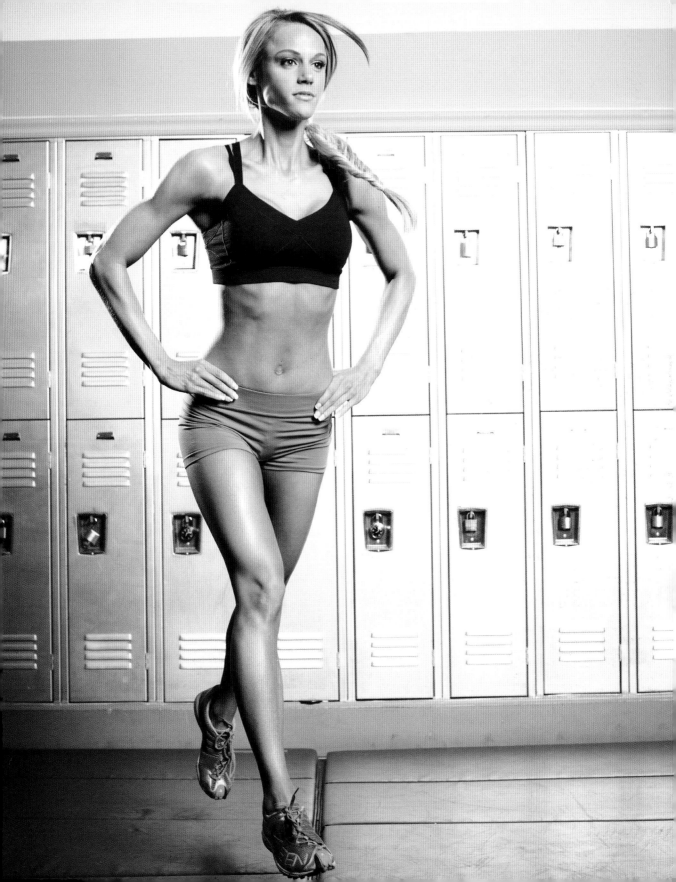

GET BACK ON TRACK

Been missing a lot of gym time lately? This four-week program will help you right the ship and improve your body in all the right places.

Okay, so it's been a while since you've been to the gym. Your body isn't exactly in the shape you'd like it to be and it's time to do something about it—quickly. Enter the following four-week program that was designed especially for women who, for whatever reason, have been inactive with hopes of getting back on track. For those who have never lifted before, detailed descriptions and photographs for each exercise are included. For those with prior experience, consider this a refresher course. Whatever your situation, your starting point to reclaiming your body is right here.

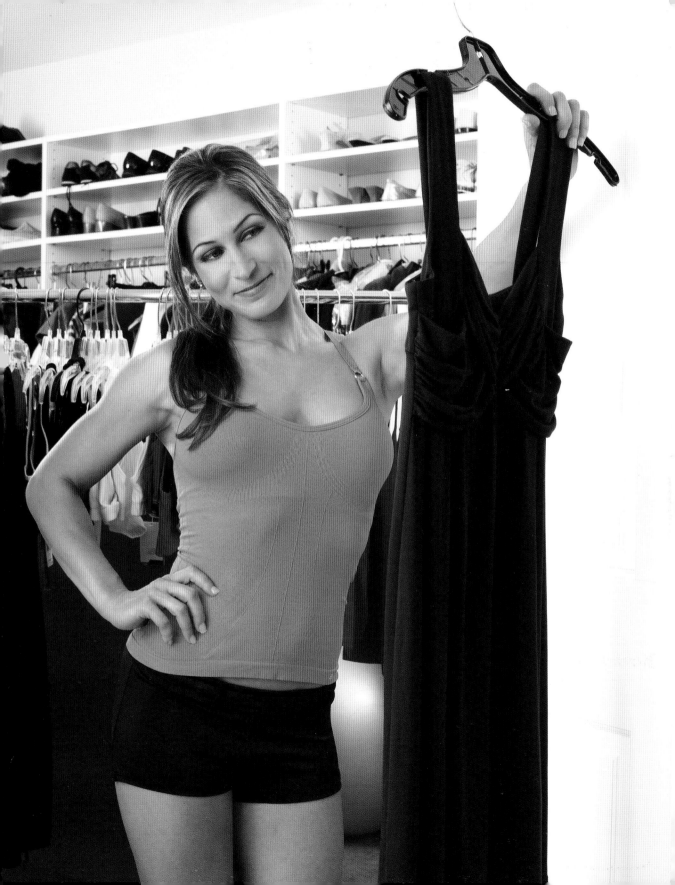

Weight Training

The lifting portion of the program is set up as a two-day, upper-/lower-body split. This means you'll train your entire body over the course of two days, and you'll do that twice a week for a total of four weekly lifting workouts. On Days 1 and 3, you'll train your major upper-body muscle groups: chest, back, shoulders, triceps, and biceps. On Days 2 and 4, you'll train your lower body: quads, glutes, hamstrings, and calves, as well as abs.

Everyone's work and family schedule is different, so if training Monday, Tuesday, Thursday, and Friday works best for you, great. If it's more convenient for you to train Sunday through Wednesday, that's fine, too.

In the first two weeks of the program, you'll do 2–3 sets and 12–15 reps of every exercise, except calves and abs, which tend to respond better to higher-rep schemes. Select a weight that allows you to reach muscle failure within the prescribed rep range. In other words, if you're able to do more than 15 reps in a set, increase the weight for your next set; if you can't do 12 reps, you'll need to lighten the load.

In Weeks 3–4, volume (total number of sets) increases to 3–4 sets per exercise, and reps decrease to 8–12. This change in rep range requires that you use a heavier weight for the last two weeks than you used for the first two. By the end of the program, you should be not only more firm throughout your body but physically stronger, as well. This newfound strength will serve a functional purpose in everyday activities and athletic endeavors.

The exercises we selected are all basic movements that have been proven effective time and again. To train legs, for example, you'll do Smith machine squats, lunges, and leg presses as your major moves; for chest, you'll do incline and bench presses and flyes. Feel free, however, to substitute exercises—barbell incline presses for dumbbell inclines, for example, or T-bar rows for seated cable rows.

INCLINE DUMBBELL PRESS

Lie faceup on an incline bench set to 45 degrees. Holding a pair of dumbbells just outside and over your shoulders, press them straight up toward the ceiling until your elbows are extended but not locked out. Slowly lower the weights back to the start position.

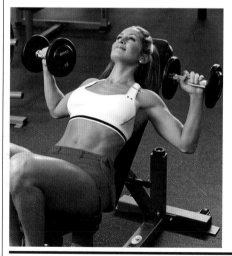

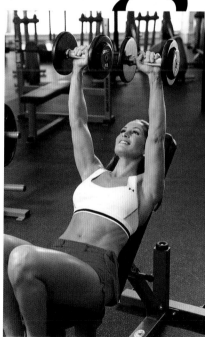

FLAT-BENCH DUMBBELL FLYE

Lie faceup on a flat bench holding a pair of relatively light dumbbells. Extend your arms over your chest, palms facing each other. With a slight bend in your elbows, lower the weights in an arc out to your sides until you feel a good stretch in your pecs. Contract your chest muscles to return the dumbbells to the start position. Keep your elbows slightly bent.

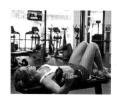

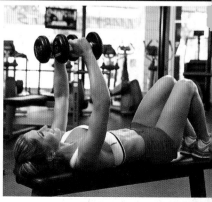

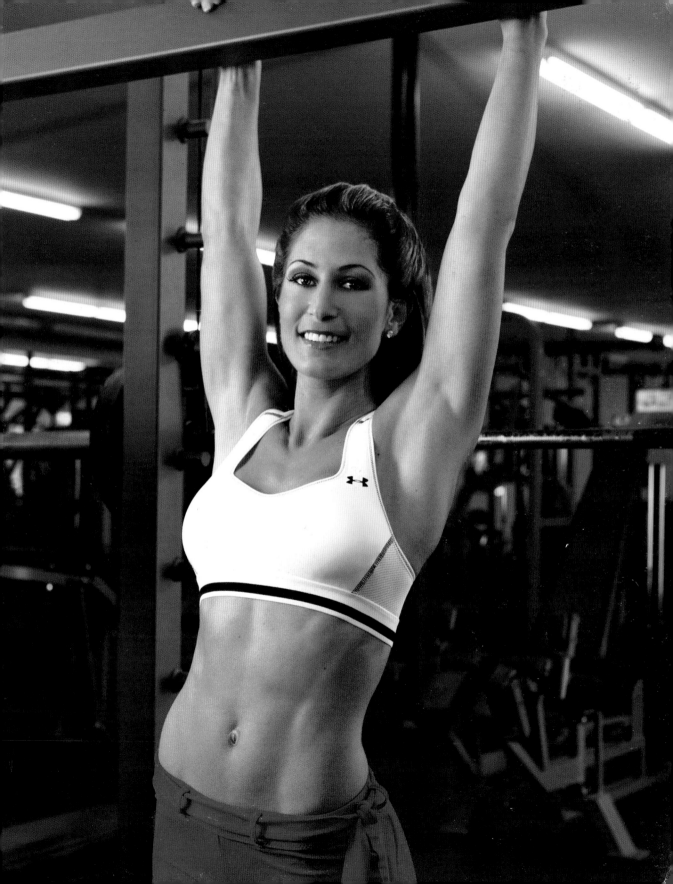

Burn F

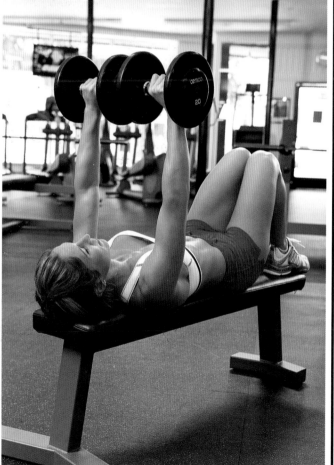

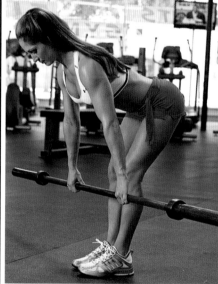

BENTOVER ROW
Stand erect holding a barbell with a shoulder-width, overhand grip. Keeping your knees slightly bent, bend at the waist until your torso is roughly parallel to the floor. Let the bar hang straight down toward the floor, arms extended. Bend your elbows and contract your back muscles to pull the bar up to your abs, keeping your torso stationary and your elbows pulled in. Squeeze at the top, then slowly lower the bar back to the arms-extended position.

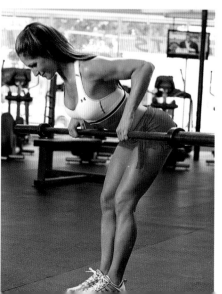

FLAT-BENCH DUMBBELL PRESS
Lie faceup on a flat bench holding a pair of dumbbells. With your elbows pointing out to your sides and the weights just outside your shoulders, press them straight up toward the ceiling until your elbows are just short of lockout. Slowly lower the dumbbells back to the start.

at

Research shows that if you do cardio before you lift weights, your weight training will suffer, so we recommend that you run, bike, or step *after* you lift. If your schedule doesn't allow you enough time to do both lifting and cardio in the same session, split them up so you do cardio in the morning before work and lift weights after work, for example.

Each cardio session will be one of two basic workouts: a steady-state session, in which intensity remains constant, or interval cardio, where you'll alternate bouts of high intensity (sprinting) with low intensity (walking). Do the steady-state sessions on lower-body lifting days since your legs will be less able to perform high-intensity cardio. You'll do intervals on upper-body days, so even after a full lifting session your legs will be fresh and ready to train intensely.

In Weeks 1 and 2, steady-state sessions will last 30 minutes (on the cardio equipment of your choice) and interval sessions will last 25 minutes, including warmup and cooldown jogs. During Weeks 3 and 4, you'll increase your cardio volume just as you do for lifting; steady-state sessions will be 45 minutes and intervals will last 35 minutes.

When it comes to your high-intensity bouts on interval days, use common sense. If it has been a few months or more since you last ran, doing all-out sprints may not be the best idea, as muscle strains and pulls are common when your legs aren't in shape. Simply run as fast as is comfortable.

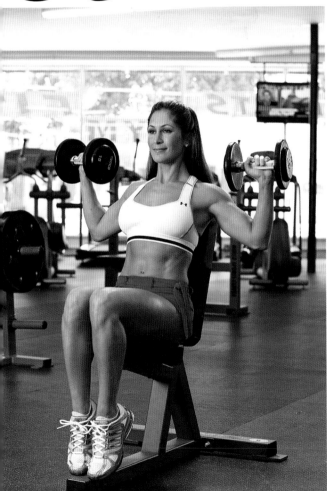

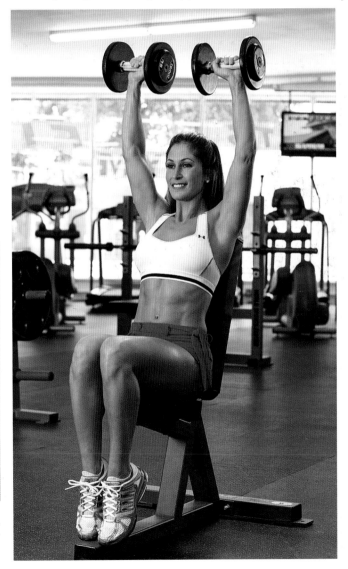

OVERHEAD DUMBBELL PRESS
Sit on a low-back seat or an adjustable bench set upright, holding a pair of dumbbells. Lift the weights to just outside your shoulders, palms facing forward. Press the dumbbells straight up until they're overhead with your elbows just short of lockout. Slowly return to the start.

What

SEATED ROW
Sit upright and place you feet flat on the platform. Keeping your knees slightly bent, lean forwar to grasp the close-grip handle, then lean back until your arms are fully extended. Contract your back muscles to pull the handle toward your mid-section, leading with you elbows. Squeeze your shoulder blades together for a count, then slowly return to start.

By the end of the four-week program your body should be feeling (and looking) better than it has in months, or even years. Now what? The key to any long-term exercise routine is consistency and progression. In other words, keep going. If you finish the program on a Friday, get right back in the gym the following Monday. At that point, it'll be time to challenge yourself even further. *Hers 360* contains tons of new workouts that'll keep your body guessing and improving, so give each of them a try. Tweaking three of the basic components of the following program—exercise selection, volume, and rep ranges—will keep you moving forward, as well.

The exercise component is easy to shake up: Simply start introducing new exercises into your training. For example, periodically substitute body-weight or assisted pullups for lat pulldowns, barbell squats for Smith machine squats, decline dumbbell presses for flat-bench presses, and so

on. The possibilities are virtually endless.

If you're ready for more of a challenge where volume is concerned, star doing more sets per muscle group. If, for instance, you could do eight total sets (four sets of two exercises) for large muscle groups, increase that to 10 sets.

As for rep ranges, this program employs mostly sets of 12–15 and 8–12. After you have four weeks under your belt, experiment with higher-rep sets (15–20), and even sets of 6–8 reps, if your goal is to increase strength. The key here is variety; don't let your muscles grow accustomed to any one-rep range.

If you stick to this program for four weeks, you'll have established a great foundation on which to build. From there, the sky's the limit. Sure, everyone gets off track now and then, but now it's time to get back on.

Next?

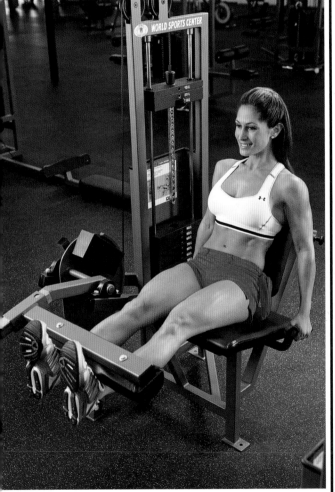

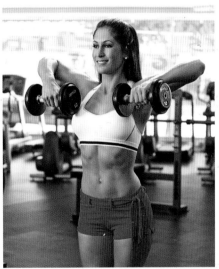

DUMBBELL UPRIGHT ROW

Stand erect holding dumbbells in front of your thighs with your hands shoulder-width apart. With your arms extended toward the floor, bend your elbows and contract your delts to lift the weights straight up along your body until they reach shoulder level. Hold for a count, then slowly lower back to the start.

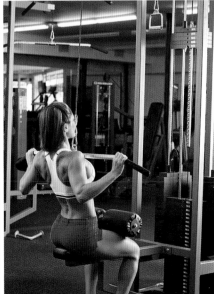

LAT PULLDOWN

Grasp the bar with an overhand grip outside shoulder width and sit down, making sure the pads fit snugly over your thighs. Begin with your arms extended overhead. Contract your lats and bend your elbows to pull the bar down in front of your face until it touches your upper chest. Squeeze for a count, then slowly return to the start position.

LEG EXTENSION

Adjust the seat so your lower back is flush with the backpad and your knees line up with the machine's axis of rotation. With your knees bent 90 degrees, lift the weight a few inches off the stack. Contract your quads to extend your knees until your legs are completely straight. Squeeze your quads for 1–2 counts at the top, then return to the start position.

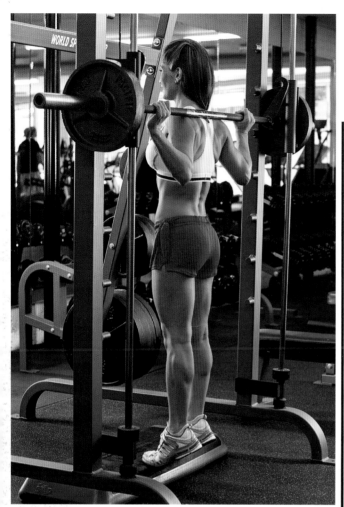

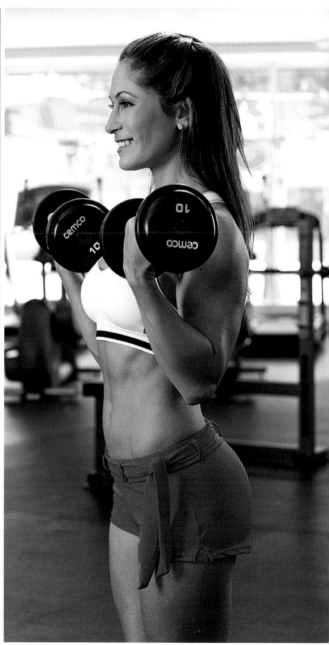

SMITH MACHINE STANDING CALF RAISE
Step onto a step on the balls of your feet, letting your heels hang off the edge. With your knees slightly bent, position your shoulders under the bar. Flex your calves to raise your ankles as high as possible. Squeeze your calves at the top, then lower back to the start, feeling a stretch at the bottom.

Back-On-Track Workout Plan
DAY 1: UPPER BODY

EXERCISE	WEEKS 1–2 SETS	REPS	WEEKS 3–4 SETS	REPS
CHEST				
Incline Dumbbell Press	2–3	12–15	3–4	8–12
Flat-bench Dumbbell Flye	2–3	12–15	3–4	8–12
BACK				
Seated Row	2–3	12–15	3–4	8–12
SHOULDERS				
Overhead Dumbbell Press	2–3	12–15	3–4	8–12
Lateral Raise	2–3	12–15	3–4	8–12
TRICEPS				
Dumbbell Lying Triceps Extension	2–3	12–15	3–4	8–12
BICEPS				
Dumbbell Curl	2–3	12–15	3–4	8–12

CARDIO (INTERVALS)
Weeks 1–2: On a treadmill or outdoors, do a five-minute warmup jog, followed by 15 minutes of "30-seconds-on, 1-minute-off" intervals, during which you sprint for 30 seconds and then walk for a minute. Finish with a five-minute cooldown jog.
Weeks 3–4: On a treadmill or outdoors, do a five-minute warmup jog, followed by 25 minutes of "30-seconds-on, 1-minute-off" intervals. Finish with a five-minute cooldown jog.

DUMBBELL CURL
Stand holding a pair of dumbbells at your sides with your arms extended toward the floor, your palms facing in and your knees slightly bent. Keeping your elbows close to your sides, curl the weights up and turn your wrists so your palms face you at the top of the rep. Squeeze for a count, then slowly lower back to the start.

ROMANIAN DEADLIFT

Stand upright holding a barbell in front of your thighs with a shoulder-width, overhand grip. Keeping your back flat and knees slightly bent, bend at the waist to lower the bar straight toward the floor, sliding it down your legs. Keep your knees slightly bent and your arms straight throughout the movement. When the bar reaches about mid-shin, contract your hamstrings and glutes to pull yourself back up to the start position.

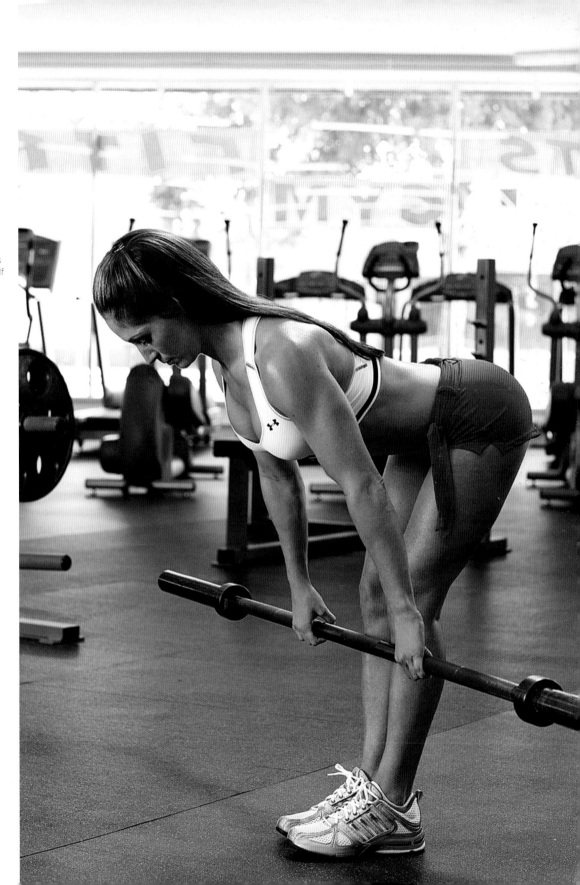

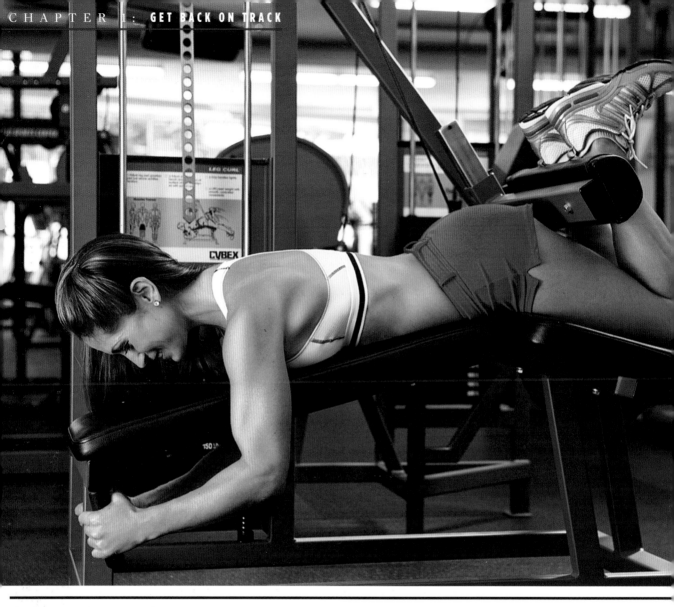

DAY 2: LOWER BODY

EXERCISE	WEEKS 1-2		WEEKS 3-4	
	SETS	REPS	SETS	REPS
QUADS/GLUTES/HAMSTRINGS				
Smith Machine Squat	2-3	12-15	3-4	8-12
QUADS				
Leg Extension	2-3	12-15	3-4	8-12
HAMSTRINGS				
Lying Leg Curl	2-3	12-15	3-4	8-12
CALVES				
Smith Machine Standing Calf Raise	2-3	15-20	3-4	12-15
ABS				
Crunch	2-3	15-20	3-4	20-25

CARDIO (STEADY STATE)

Weeks 1-2: 30 minutes at 60%-65% of your max heart rate (220 minus your age, multiplied by 0.6 and 0.65) on the cardio equipment of your choice (treadmill, stair-stepper, elliptical trainer, stationary bike, etc.)

Weeks 3-4: 45 minutes at 65%-80% of your max heart rate (220 minus your age, multiplied by 0.65 and 0.8) on the cardio equipment of your choice

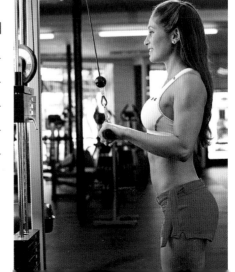

PRESSDOWN
Attach a straight bar, EZ bar or rope to a high-pulley cable. Stand facing the stack and grasp the attachment with both hands, keeping your elbows in tight to your sides and your upper arms just above parallel to the floor. Press the bar or rope toward the floor until your arms are fully extended. Squeeze your triceps at the bottom, then slowly return to the start.

LYING LEG CURL

Adjust the machine so the roller pad fits over the backs of your ankles. Lie facedown on the bench and grasp the handles for stability. Start with your legs straight and the weight lifted a few inches off the stack. Bend your knees to curl your lower legs toward your glutes without lifting your thighs. Squeeze your hamstrings for a count, then slowly lower to the start.

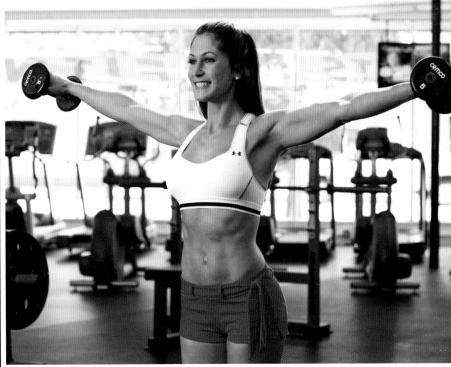

LATERAL RAISE

Stand erect holding a pair of light dumbbells in a neutral grip about four inches away from your sides with your knees and elbows slightly bent. Keeping your elbows fixed, lift the weights up and out to your sides until your arms are just past parallel to the floor. Hold for a brief count, then slowly lower the dumbbells back to the start position.

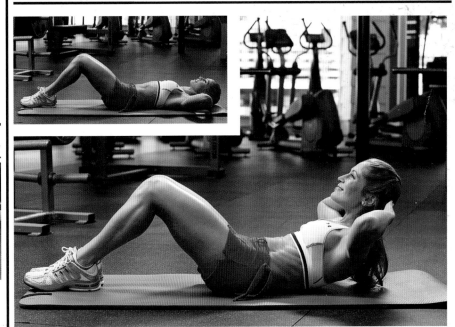

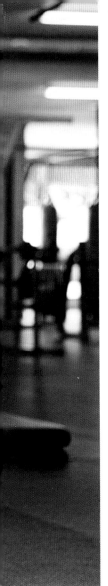

REVERSE CRUNCH

Lie faceup on the floor with your hands under your hips. Lift your legs off the floor and bend your knees 90 degrees so your lower legs are parallel to the floor. Contract your abs to pull your pelvis toward your ribcage, and raise your glutes and lower back off the floor. Squeeze for a count at the top, then slowly lower back to the start position.

CRUNCH

Lie faceup on the floor with your knees bent and your feet flat on the floor. Either cross your arms over your chest or cup your hands lightly behind your head. Contract your abs to lift your shoulder blades 6–12 inches off the floor, then slowly lower yourself back down. The range of motion is very small.

DAY 3: UPPER BODY

EXERCISE	WEEKS 1-2 SETS	WEEKS 1-2 REPS	WEEKS 3-4 SETS	WEEKS 3-4 REPS
BACK				
Bentover Row	2-3	12-15	3-4	8-12
Lat Pulldown	2-3	12-15	3-4	8-12
CHEST				
Flat-bench Dumbbell Press	2-3	12-15	3-4	8-12
SHOULDERS				
Dumbbell Upright Row	2-3	12-15	3-4	8-12
BICEPS				
Cable Curl	2-3	12-15	3-4	8-12
TRICEPS				
Pressdown	2-3	12-15	3-4	8-12

CARDIO (INTERVALS)

Weeks 1–2: On a treadmill or outdoors, do a five-minute warmup jog, followed by 15 minutes of "1-minute-on, 1-minute-off" intervals, where you sprint for a minute and then walk for a minute. Finish with a five-minute cooldown jog.

Weeks 3–4: On a treadmill or outdoors, do a five-minute warmup jog, followed by 25 minutes of "30-seconds-on, 1-minute-off" intervals. Finish with a five-minute cooldown jog.

DAY 4: LOWER BODY

EXERCISE	WEEKS 1-2 SETS	WEEKS 1-2 REPS	WEEKS 3-4 SETS	WEEKS 3-4 REPS
QUADS/GLUTES/HAMSTRINGS				
Dumbbell Lunge	2-3	12-15	3-4	8-12
Leg Press	2-3	12-15	3-4	8-12
HAMSTRINGS				
Romanian Deadlift	2-3	12-15	3-4	8-12
CALVES				
Seated Calf Raise	2-3	15-20	3-4	12-15
ABS				
Reverse Crunch	2-3	15-20	3-4	20-25

CARDIO (STEADY STATE)

Weeks 1–2: 30 minutes at 60%–65% of your max heart rate (220 minus your age, multiplied by 0.6 and 0.65) on the cardio equipment of your choice (treadmill, stair-stepper, elliptical trainer, stationary bike)

Weeks 3–4: 45 minutes at 65%–80% of your max heart rate (220 minus your age, multiplied by 0.65 and 0.8) on the cardio equipment of your choice

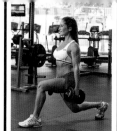

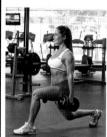

DUMBBELL LUNGE

Stand erect with your feet together, holding a dumbbell in each hand with your arms at your sides. Take a big step forward with one leg, landing heel first. Bend that knee and your back knee to lower yourself toward the floor. Before your trailing knee touches down, push back up with your front leg to return to the start. Alternate legs.

CABLE CURL

Attach a straight bar to a low-pulley cable and stand a couple of feet away from the weight stack. Take a shoulder-width, underhand grip and extend your arms straight down in front of you. Bend your knees slightly to relieve pressure on your lower back. Keeping your elbows pinned at your sides, curl the bar as high as you can. Squeeze your biceps at the top, then slowly return to the start.

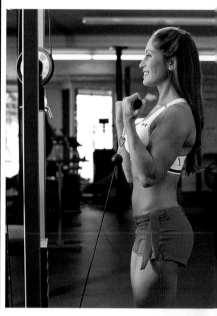

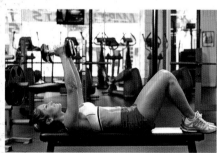

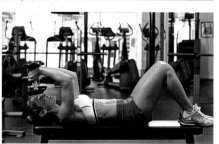

DUMBBELL LYING TRICEPS EXTENSION

Lie faceup on a flat bench and hold dumbbells with a neutral grip. Lift the weights directly above you until your arms are extended and perpendicular to the floor. Keeping your upper arms stationary, slowly lower the weights toward your forehead. At the bottom, contract your triceps and press the dumbbells back up to the start position.

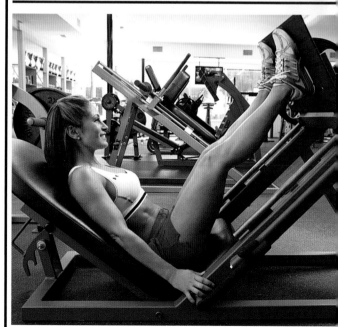

LEG PRESS

Sit in a leg-press machine and place your feet hip- to shoulder-width apart in the middle of the platform above you. Press up until your knees are just short of lockout. Release the machine's safety catches, and lower the sled under control until your knees form 90-degree angles. Push back up explosively to the start.

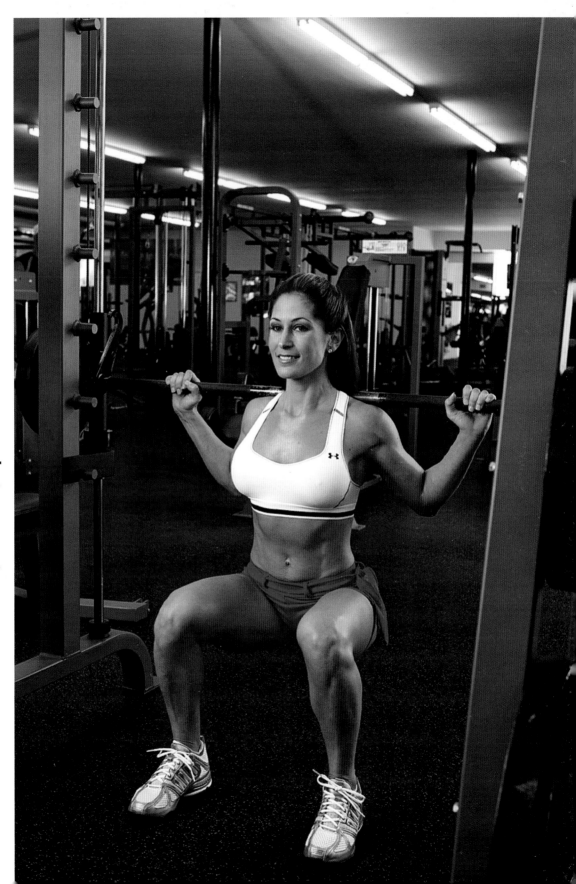

SMITH MACHINE SQUAT

Stand under the bar so it rests across your traps, grasping it to keep it stable. With your feet about shoulder-width apart and a foot in front of the bar, keep your head straight and eyes forward, and push your chest out slightly so your back naturally arches. Release the safety hooks and squat as if to sit in a chair, keeping your feet in full contact with the floor and maintaining the arch in your back. When your thighs come parallel to the floor, push up through your heels, extending your knees and hips to return to the standing position.

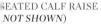

SEATED CALF RAISE (NOT SHOWN)

Sit on the seat and adjust the pads so they fit snugly over your lower thighs. Place the balls of your feet and toes on the platform so your heels are suspended. Release the safety catch and begin with your heels below the level of the platform so you feel a stretch in your calves. Extend your ankles to push the pads toward the ceiling as high as you can—you should be almost on tiptoe at the top. Squeeze your calves, then lower back down.

CHAPTER 2

SPLIT DECISION

Deciding which body parts to train together can be a real puzzle.
We solve it for you.

To make noticeable improvements in your physique over weeks and months, you need to know how to change up your training. Whether through variables such as exercise and weight selection, sets and reps, or even your rest periods between sets, continually tweaking your workouts helps stave off plateaus and keeps the beneficial muscular adaptations coming. But before you can even consider altering your training variables, you need to decide on your training split. The split you use determines how frequently you work out each week, how often you exercise each muscle group in a week and what body parts get trained together.

Your current split may be something you adopted from a training partner or lifted from a popular fitness competitor's split presented in *Hers.* While it may be good, it may not be the best split for you.

And even if it's a great split, you should change it up from time to time as you do other training variables to prompt the gains you're looking for.

Why? For one thing, if you keep your training split the same month after month, your muscles will adapt and get stale, limiting your progress. Two, if you train the same body parts in the same order every time, the muscles you hit later in the routine can't be worked with the same intensity as the ones trained first, again limiting your results.

While an endless combination of training splits exist, several fit a variety of experience levels and schedules. Here we lay out the four most common splits, and in the "Trial Separation" section we provide a way for you to try them all over the course of 12 weeks to help you gauge which ones work better for you.

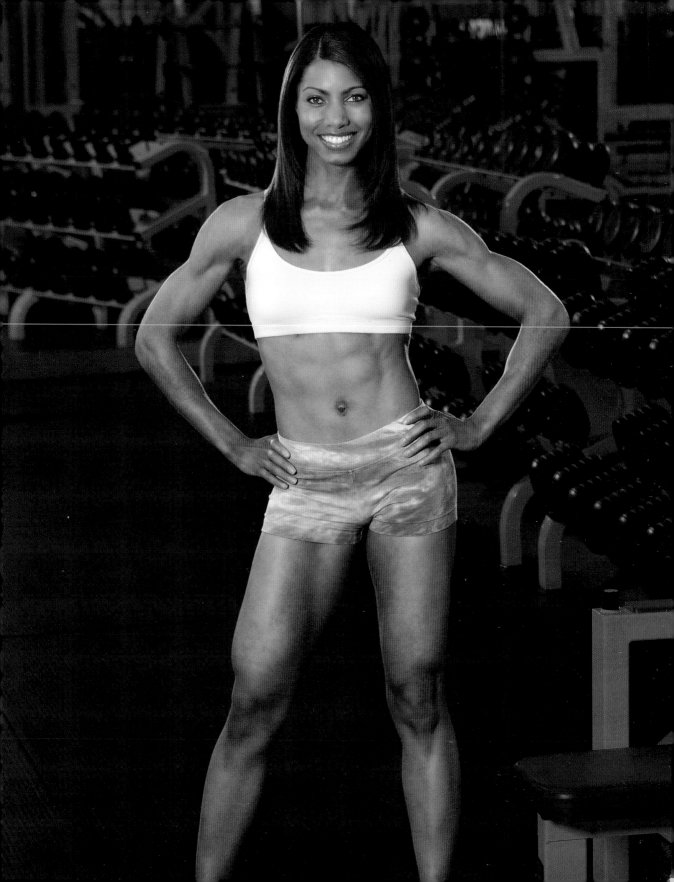

SPLIT No.1

WHOLE BODY
(THREE DAYS PER WEEK)

Here you simply train the entire body each time you go to the gym. Typically, most whole-body workouts use only 1–2 exercises per muscle group with total sets per body part rarely exceeding six. This allows you to train each muscle group more frequently because it receives a limited amount of stress in each workout. The less stress a muscle receives, the faster it can recover and be ready for your next training session.

Although typically considered a beginner split, the whole-body option can also work well for advanced lifters. Training such a large number of muscle groups in each workout boosts growth hormone levels, which helps to encourage muscle growth as well as fat burning. Whole-body training also activates a greater amount of enzymes in muscles that turn on fat-burning processes.

In addition, research from St. Francis Xavier University (Antigonish, Nova Scotia, Canada) showed that female and male subjects who trained each muscle group three times per week had upper-body strength gains 8% greater and muscle mass gains 300% greater than those who trained twice a week. This was despite the fact that each group completed the same number of sets per muscle group, which means the three-times-per-week trainees did fewer sets per workout. So if you currently train each body part once a week for about 12 sets each, training each muscle group with four sets three times a week on a whole-body split instead will allow you to do the same number of sets per week but may enhance your results.

The simplest way to use the whole-body approach is to train on Monday, Wednesday, and Friday, thus allowing at least one full day of rest between workouts. Of course, any three days that provide at least one day of rest between workouts will do, such as a Tuesday, Thursday, and Saturday schedule. Be sure to do a different exercise for every muscle group in each of the three workouts per week to avoid staleness, and alternate the order of the muscle groups you train, being sure to move weak body parts earlier in the workout on some days. Our sample program accomplishes both of these goals to optimize your results.

MONDAY

MUSCLE GROUP	EXERCISE	SETS/REPS
Chest	Incline Dumbbell Flye	4/10–12
Shoulders	Upright Row	4/10–12
Triceps	Pressdown	4/10–12
Quads	Leg Extension	3/10–12
Back	Lat Pulldown	4/10–12
Biceps	Incline Dumbbell Curl	4/10–12
Hams	Lying Leg Curl	3/10–12
Abs	Reverse Crunch	4/12–15
Calves	Standing Calf Raise	4/10–12

WEDNESDAY

MUSCLE GROUP	EXERCISE	SETS/REPS
Quads/Hams/Glutes	Squat	4/6–8
Chest	Dumbbell Press	4/6–8
Back	Seated Cable Row	4/6–8
Shoulders	Overhead Dumbbell Press	4/6–8
Biceps	Barbell Curl	4/6–8
Triceps	Lying Triceps Extension	4/6–8
Calves	Seated Calf Raise	4/12–15
Abs	Hanging Leg Raise	4/10–12

FRIDAY

MUSCLE GROUP	EXERCISE	SETS/REPS
Back	Barbell Row	4/15–20
Biceps	Preacher Curl	4/15–20
Quads/Hams/Glutes	Dumbbell Lunge	4/15–20
Calves	Leg Press Calf Raise	4/15–20
Chest	Cable Crossover	4/15–20
Shoulders	Lateral Raise	4/15–20
Triceps	Overhead Triceps Extension	4/15–20
Abs	Crunch	4/15–20

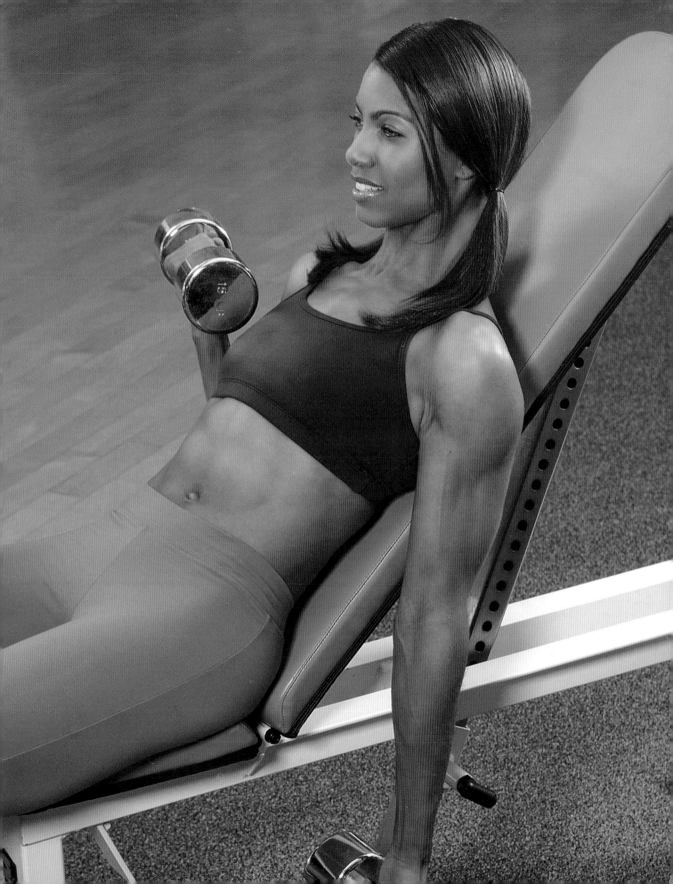

SPLIT No. 2

UPPER/ LOWER BODY

(FOUR DAYS PER WEEK)

In this split you break the body into upper (chest, back, shoulders, biceps, and triceps) and lower (quads, hams, calves, glutes, and abs) muscle groups. You can train each body part twice weekly, in two upper-body and two lower-body workouts.

Because you split the entire body into two workouts, you can do more sets for each muscle group than in the whole-body split. It also allows you to train with a little more intensity, since you have fewer muscle groups to focus on each time you visit the gym. Yet because this type of split allows for more sets and higher intensity, it means your muscles will require more rest. Most people who follow an upper/lower split follow a standard Monday (lower-body workout 1), Tuesday (upper-body workout 1), Thursday (lower-body workout 2), and Friday (upper-body workout 2) training schedule as shown. This allows each muscle group two full days of rest between workouts.

SPLITTING THE DIFFERENCES

Follow the program schedule in "Trial Separation" (page 28), using each training split for three weeks. This will give you just enough time to get a feel for each one and determine how well your body responds, as well as how well it works with your schedule. These are all-important considerations. We also give you questions to help you grade the benefits of the various splits.

Regardless of which split you find works best for you, you'll still want to consider swapping it out every once in a while. For example, if you find that the four-day split is your No. 1 choice, use it for a good portion of the year, but every 3–4 months switch to a different training split for at least a month or two.

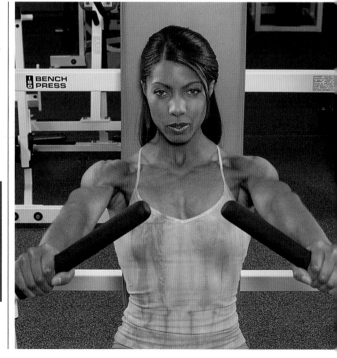

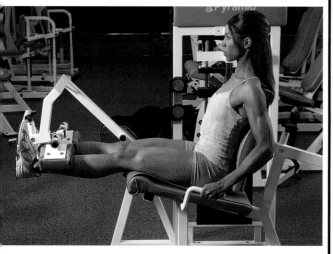

ONDAY (LOWER BODY)

MUSCLE GROUP	EXERCISE	SETS/REPS
uads/Hams/Glutes	Squat	4/8–10
uads	Leg Extension	3/12–15
amstrings	Lying Leg Curl	3/10–12
alves	Leg Press Calf Raise	3/15–20
	Seated Calf Raise	3/20–25
bs	Hanging Leg Raise	3/10–12
	Crunch	3/15–20

UESDAY (UPPER BODY)

MUSCLE GROUP	EXERCISE	SETS/REPS
hest	Incline Dumbbell Press	3/6–8
	Dumbbell Flye	3/8–10
ack	Lat Pulldown	3/8–10
	Seated Cable Row	3/10–12
houlders	Overhead Dumbbell Press	3/8–10
	Lateral Raise	2/12–15
riceps	Pressdown	2/10–12
	Lying Triceps Extension	2/12–15
iceps	Barbell Curl	2/10–12
	Preacher Curl	2/12–15

HURSDAY (LOWER BODY)

MUSCLE GROUP	EXERCISE	SETS/REPS
uads/Hams/Glutes	Dumbbell Lunge	3/10–12
ams/Glutes	Romanian Deadlift	3/8–10
uads	Leg Extension	3/12–15
alves	Seated Calf Raise	3/15–20
	Standing Calf Raise	3/15–20
bs	Cable Crunch	3/10–12
	Reverse Crunch	3/15–20

RIDAY (UPPER BODY)

MUSCLE GROUP	EXERCISE	SETS/REPS
ack	Barbell Row	3/8–10
	Reverse-grip Pulldown	3/10–12
iceps	Incline Dumbbell Curl	2/8–10
	Cable Curl	2/10–12
hest	Machine Chest Press	3/10–12
	Incline Dumbbell Flye	3/12–15
houlders	Upright Row	2/10–12
	Bentover Lateral Raise	2/15–20
riceps	Overhead Triceps Extension	2/8–10
	Kickback	2/10–12

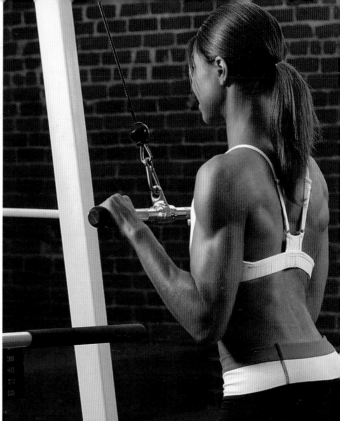

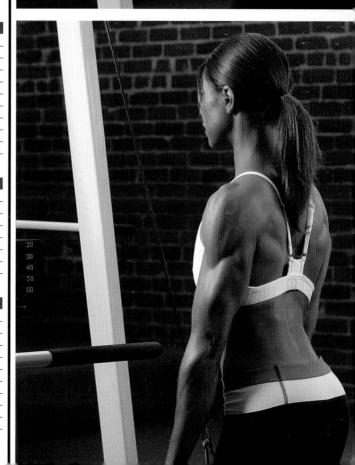

SPLIT No.3

PUSH/ PULL/ LEGS
(THREE DAYS PER WEEK)

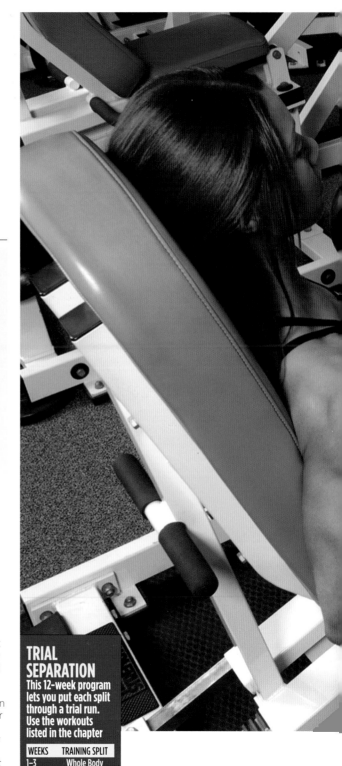

The push/pull/legs split is based on the concept that the body's muscles are mainly divided into pushing and pulling muscles. Pushing muscles include the chest, shoulders, and triceps, which tend to push the weight away from the body, such as during the bench press, overhead press, and triceps extension. Pulling muscles include the back and biceps, which mainly pull the weight toward the body, such as during barbell rows and dumbbell curls. Abs are commonly considered pulling muscles because they pull the torso toward the legs and/or the legs toward the torso.

The problem arises when you consider legs. The squat is a pushing exercise, as is the leg extension, but moves such as leg curls and Romanian deadlifts are pulling exercises. But the issue is resolved by giving legs their own training day.

Because the entire body is trained over three separate workouts, many people who follow this split train on Monday, Wednesday, and Friday, hitting each muscle group once a week. Yet some do it six days a week to hit each body part twice over the seven-day span. We suggest the former to prevent overtraining.

TRIAL SEPARATION
This 12-week program lets you put each split through a trial run. Use the workouts listed in the chapter

WEEKS	TRAINING SPLIT
1–3	Whole Body
4–6	Upper Body/ Lower Body
7–9	Push/Pull/Legs
10–12	Four Day

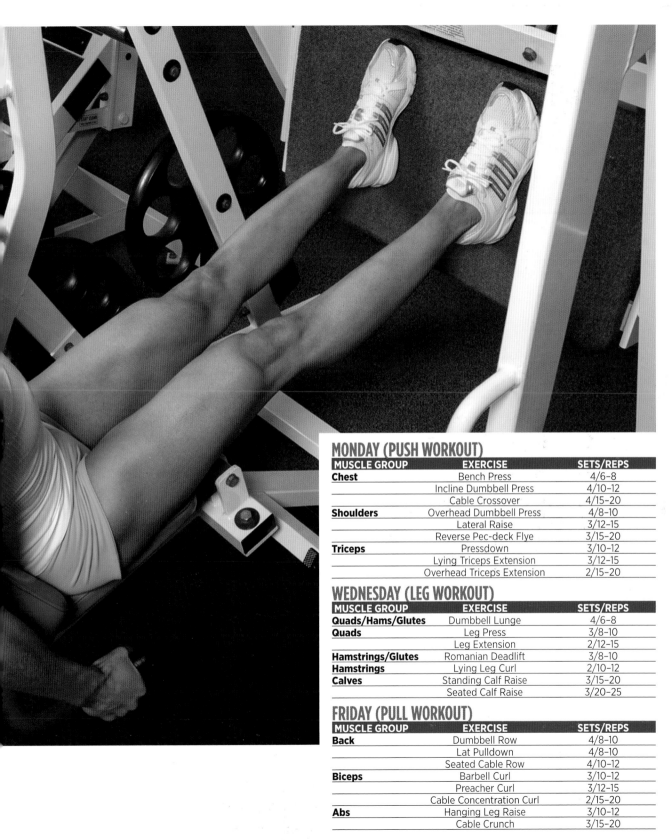

MONDAY (PUSH WORKOUT)

MUSCLE GROUP	EXERCISE	SETS/REPS
Chest	Bench Press	4/6–8
	Incline Dumbbell Press	4/10–12
	Cable Crossover	4/15–20
Shoulders	Overhead Dumbbell Press	4/8–10
	Lateral Raise	3/12–15
	Reverse Pec-deck Flye	3/15–20
Triceps	Pressdown	3/10–12
	Lying Triceps Extension	3/12–15
	Overhead Triceps Extension	2/15–20

WEDNESDAY (LEG WORKOUT)

MUSCLE GROUP	EXERCISE	SETS/REPS
Quads/Hams/Glutes	Dumbbell Lunge	4/6–8
Quads	Leg Press	3/8–10
	Leg Extension	2/12–15
Hamstrings/Glutes	Romanian Deadlift	3/8–10
Hamstrings	Lying Leg Curl	2/10–12
Calves	Standing Calf Raise	3/15–20
	Seated Calf Raise	3/20–25

FRIDAY (PULL WORKOUT)

MUSCLE GROUP	EXERCISE	SETS/REPS
Back	Dumbbell Row	4/8–10
	Lat Pulldown	4/8–10
	Seated Cable Row	4/10–12
Biceps	Barbell Curl	3/10–12
	Preacher Curl	3/12–15
	Cable Concentration Curl	2/15–20
Abs	Hanging Leg Raise	3/10–12
	Cable Crunch	3/15–20

SPLIT No. 4

FOUR-DAY TRAINING
(FOUR DAYS PER WEEK)

This split simply divides all the major muscle groups of the body into four separate training days. This means you train fewer body parts per workout than the three splits we've described, allowing you to increase both the intensity of your workouts and the number of exercises and sets you perform per muscle group.

Most four-day splits are performed on a Monday, Tuesday, Thursday, Friday schedule, with rest days on Wednesday, Saturday, and Sunday. Yet you can train any four days of the week you prefer.

You can divide up muscle groups in many ways with a four-day training split, but here we've paired body parts that perform opposite actions. For example, on Monday you'll train quads, hams, calves, and abs; on Tuesday you'll do back and chest; on Thursday you'll work shoulders and abs; and on Friday it's time for biceps and triceps.

The Tuesday and Friday workouts listed here best exemplify the benefits of this training strategy. Pairing chest with back and biceps with triceps allows you to train two muscle groups that don't fatigue each other. Each body part performs an opposite motion of its pair, a push vs. a pull.

MONDAY (LEGS + ABS)

MUSCLE GROUP	EXERCISE	SETS/REPS
Quads/Hams/Glutes	Squat	4/8-10
	Step-up	3/10-15
Quads	Leg Extension	3/12-15
Hamstrings	Lying Leg Curl	3/12-15
Hams/Glutes	Romanian Deadlift	3/12-15
Calves	Standing Calf Raise	4/10-12
	Seated Calf Raise	4/12-15
Abs	Reverse Crunch	3/12-15
	Exercise Ball Crunch	3/15-20

TUESDAY (BACK + CHEST)

MUSCLE GROUP	EXERCISE	SETS/REPS
Back	Lat Pulldown	3/8-10
	Barbell Row	3/8-10
	Seated Cable Row	3/10-12
	Straight-arm Pulldown	3/10-12
Chest	Smith Machine Bench Press	3/8-10
	Incline Dumbbell Press	3/8-10
	Incline Dumbbell Flye	3/10-12
	Pec-deck or Machine Flye	3/10-12

THURSDAY (SHOULDERS + ABS)

MUSCLE GROUP	EXERCISE	SETS/REPS
Shoulders	Smith Machine Shoulder Press	3/8-10
	Smith Machine Upright Row	3/8-10
	One-arm Cable Lateral Raise	3/10-12
	Bentover Lateral Raise	3/10-12
Abs	Decline Crunch	3/12-15
	Oblique Crunch	3/12-15

FRIDAY (BICEPS + TRICEPS)

MUSCLE GROUP	EXERCISE	SETS/REPS
Biceps	Alternating Dumbbell Curl	3/8-10
	Cable Curl	3/10-12
	EZ-bar Preacher Curl	3/10-12
Triceps	Smith Close-grip Bench Press	3/8-10
	Pressdown	3/10-12
	One-arm Overhead Dumbbell Extension	3/10-12

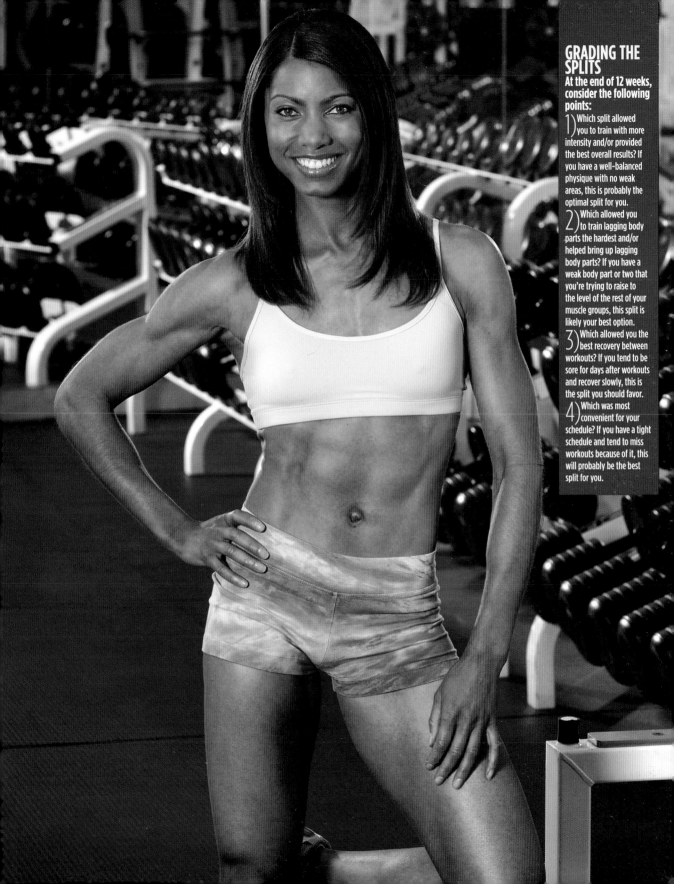

PUMP UP THE VOLUME

These six high-intensity training techniques will push your workouts, and your physique, to the next level

You've just come to the very last rep you can manage on that challenging set of squats, presses, or whatever exercise you happen to be doing. This is your last rep and your muscles are spent, so the set's over, right? Wrong. There's still more to do. Don't stop just yet.

Why keep going when your muscles have already been taken to failure and you can very easily end the set and be in good shape? Because if you keep pushing past failure using the following high-intensity training tips, you'll be even better off in terms of muscle size, strength, and definition. Consider these six techniques exactly what your muscles need to reach their full potential.

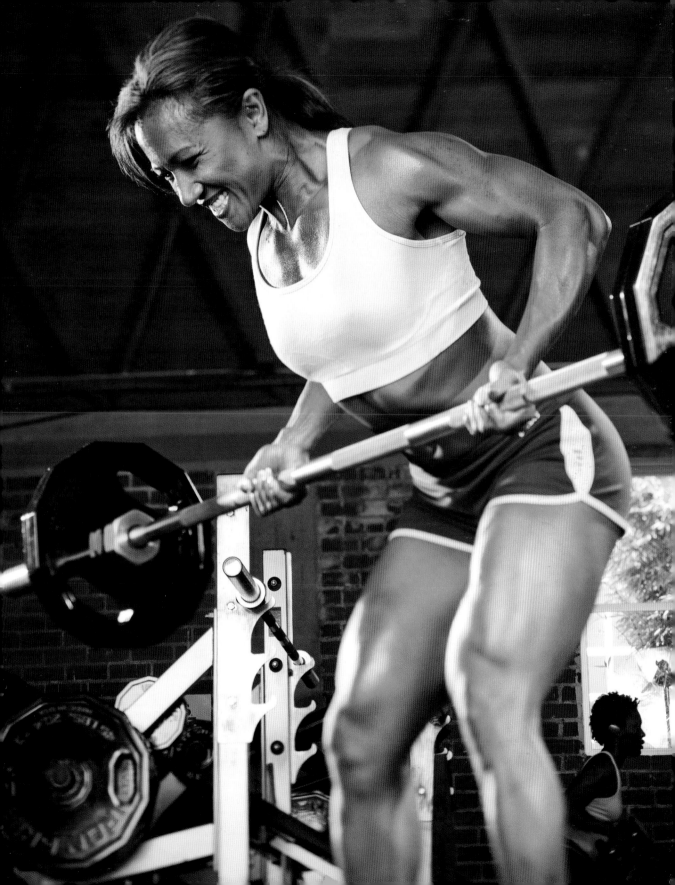

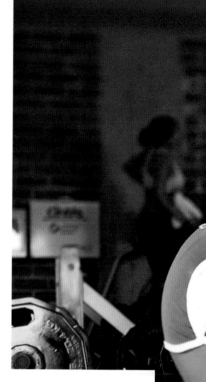

Supersets

WHAT IT IS: One set each of two different exercises performed back to back with no rest in between. A superset can consist of moves for different body parts (such as chest and back or quads and shoulders) or the same muscle group (like two biceps exercises).

WHY DO IT: To boost training intensity and do more work in less time. When supersetting different body parts, one rests while you train the other, so you can essentially cut your rest time in half. Using chest and back as an example, your back recovers when you do presses; when you do rows, your chest rests. Supersetting exercises for the same muscle group thoroughly exhausts that body part, which is great for bringing up a weak area and breaking through a plateau. New research has found that you burn about 35% more calories during the workout as well as afterward when you use supersets compared to standard sets. This means you'll burn more fat.

HOW TO DO IT: Opposing muscle groups (chest and back, biceps and triceps, quads and hams) are ideal for supersetting to promote muscular balance. (Not that there's anything wrong with pairing, say, shoulders and biceps.) When supersetting the same muscle group, do the more difficult exercise first. With biceps, for example, superset barbell curls and concentration curls in that order. Yet many fitness and figure pros like to do the opposite in pre-exhaust supersets such as leg extensions followed by barbell squats.

Sample Superset Back Routine

EXERCISE	SETS	REPS	REST
Pullup (or assisted pullup)	3	To failure	—
—*superset with*—			
Bentover Dumbbell Row	3	8–10	2–3 min.
Straight-arm Pulldown	3	12–15	—
—*superset with*—			
Wide-grip Lat Pulldown	3	12–15	2–3 min.

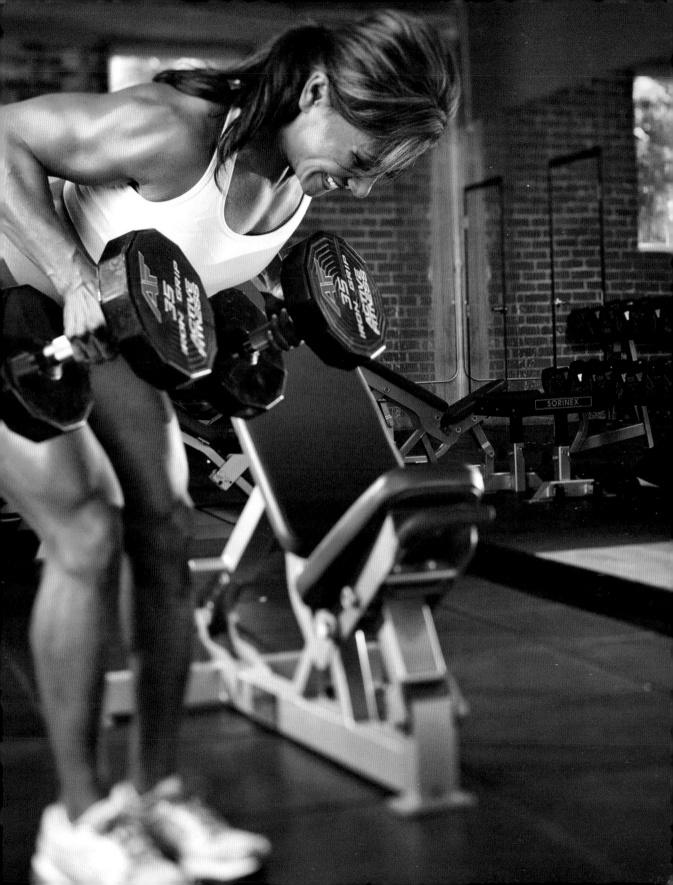

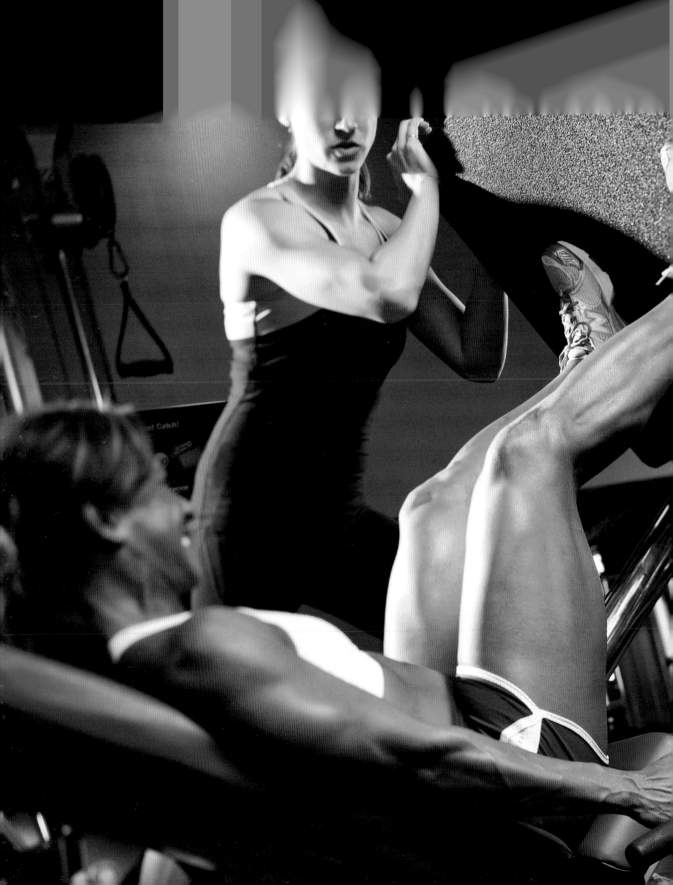

Forced Reps

WHAT IT IS: A technique in which you reach failure on a set before a spotter helps lift the weight so you can get past your sticking point and continue the set.

WHY DO IT: Research confirms that forced reps increase growth-hormone levels (GH) more than sets taken only to muscle failure. For a woman, boosting GH levels is critical for strength and muscle building, since testosterone levels are naturally low in females. GH is also essential for fat burning: It has been shown that athletes using forced reps drop more body fat than those who stop at failure.

HOW DO IT: The key to effective forced-rep training is having a spotter who knows what she's doing. The objective is to get 2–4 forced reps at the end of a set, not 8–10. For that reason, the spotter shouldn't help too much. She should make you work hard through each and every forced rep, providing just enough assistance to get you past your sticking point. That said, the spotter shouldn't make you work so hard that the reps take five seconds on the concentric portion; when doing forced reps, the weight should always keep moving. If it stops, the spotter isn't providing enough help.

Sample Forced-Reps Quad Workout

EXERCISE	SETS	REPS	REST
Leg Press	4	10–12*	2 min.
Dumbbell Lunge	4	10–12 (per leg)	2 min.
Leg Extension	3	12–15*	1–2 min.

*Perform 2–4 forced reps on your last two sets.

Dropsets

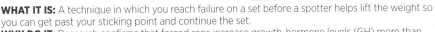

WHAT IT IS: A set in which you reach failure with the initial load, then immediately decrease the weight and do more reps to failure. The set is either finished at this point or multiple dropsets are performed, where you decrease the weight further and reach failure each time.

WHY DO IT: Dropsets allow you to take your muscles past failure on a given exercise and extend a set without resting, which increases intensity to promote gains in size and definition. If you have a weak body part that could use extra attention, dropsets are ideal.

HOW TO DO IT: Dropping the right amount of weight is key, as is exercise selection. If you don't go light enough you'll be able to do only a few more reps, if that; if you drop too much weight, your muscles won't be challenged enough to get the full benefit of the technique. If you failed at, say, 10 reps with the initial weight, you want to fail at 8–10 reps on subsequent dropsets rather than 3–5. A good rule of thumb is to decrease the weight by 20–30% on each dropset; research confirms this is the best weight range for optimal results. The best exercises for dropsets are dumbbell, machine, and cable moves, where the resistance can be decreased quickly to minimize rest. With dumbbells, picking up a lighter pair of weights takes only a few seconds. On machines and cables, moving the pin up on the weight stack is a quick change as well.

Sample Dropset Delt Routine

EXERCISE	SETS	REPS	REST
Barbell Overhead Press	4*	8	2–3 min.
Smith Machine Upright Row	3*	10–12	2 min.
Barbell Front Raise	3*	10–12	2 min.
Dumbbell Lateral Raise	3	12–15	1–2 min.

*Perform two dropsets on the last two sets.

Negatives

WHAT IT IS: An advanced method in which, with the help of a spotter, you perform only the eccentric (negative) portion of each rep at a very slow pace. Traditionally, strength athletes do negatives as stand-alone sets, but this technique can also be used at the end of a regular set to train the muscles past failure.

WHY DO IT: Negatives provide a unique shock to your muscles and are very effective at increasing strength as well as muscle growth. Most people disregard the eccentric portion of the rep, thinking the muscle works only when you lift the weight. Not true. Resisting the weight on the negative is a crucial aspect of strength and is actually the part of the movement most closely associated with muscle soreness in the days following a workout. And that soreness equates to increased size and strength.

HOW TO DO IT: The specifics of how to do negatives are crucial. First, you'll need a dependable spotter. After reaching failure on a regular set, do 2–3 negatives in this manner: Your spotter will lift the weight through the positive portion of the rep for you, then you'll lower the weight slowly for a count of 3–5 seconds. Even though you lower the weight on your own, your spotter will need to be highly attentive just in case your muscles give out and you can no longer resist the weight.

Sample Negatives Back Routine

EXERCISE	SETS	REPS	REST
Pullup (or assisted pullup)	4	8*	2–3 min.
Machine Row	3–4	10–12*	2 min.
Lat Pulldown	3	12–15	1–2 min.

Do 2–3 negatives on the last two sets.

Partial Reps

WHAT IT IS: A technique in which reps are performed short of your full range of motion (ROM), typically at the end of a set when strict reps are no longer possible due to fatigue that prevents you from lifting the weight past your "sticking point."

WHY DO IT: Because you'd rather not stop to rest, lighten the weight, or end the set just yet. Achieving full ROM is always recommended, but used occasionally, partials can help you seamlessly extend a set to fatigue your muscle fibers that much more, even if it's just in the bottom or top half of the movement.

HOW TO DO IT: When using partial reps, a majority of the set is still taken through a full ROM. Using biceps curls as an example, let's say you choose a weight you can lift for 10 strict reps. When you've reached failure and can't move the bar past a certain point (somewhere around halfway up, a common curling sticking point), simply do reps in which you lift the weight as far as possible, even if it's only a few inches as you grow more fatigued. These reps are typically done quickly, not slow and controlled, and you likely won't be able to do more than a handful of partials before the burn is unbearable and the weight won't budge an inch. Even though your ROM is limited, use proper form in other areas. For example, with curls keep your elbows pinned to your sides and don't lean back.

Sample Partial-Reps Triceps Routine

EXERCISE	SETS	REPS	REST
Lying Triceps Extension	4	8–10	2 min.
Cable Pushdown	3	10–12*	2 min.
Kickback	3	12–15*	1–2 min.

Perform partial reps at the end of your last 1–2 sets after reaching failure on full ROM reps. Do partials until you can no longer budge the weight.

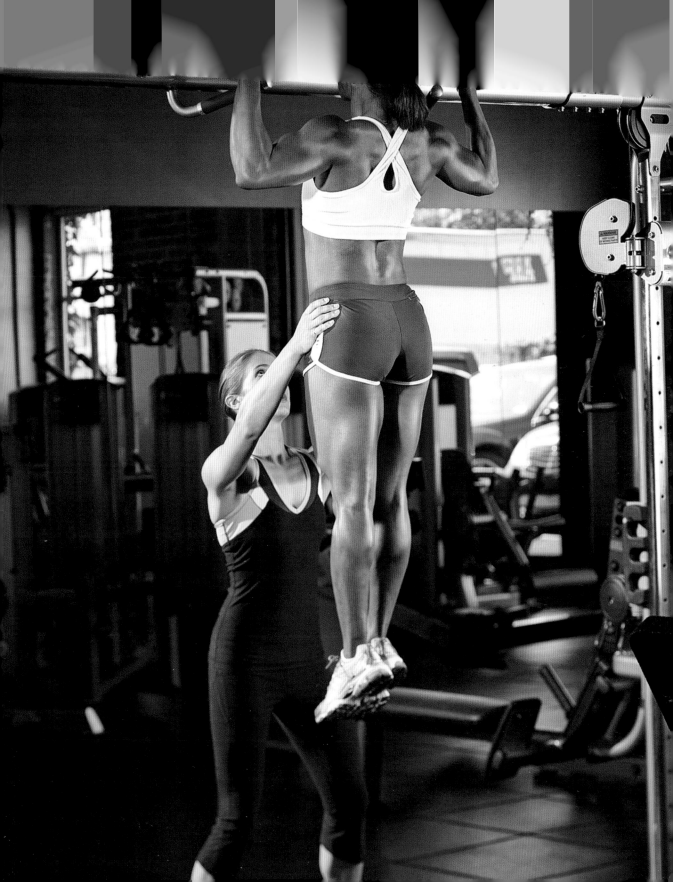

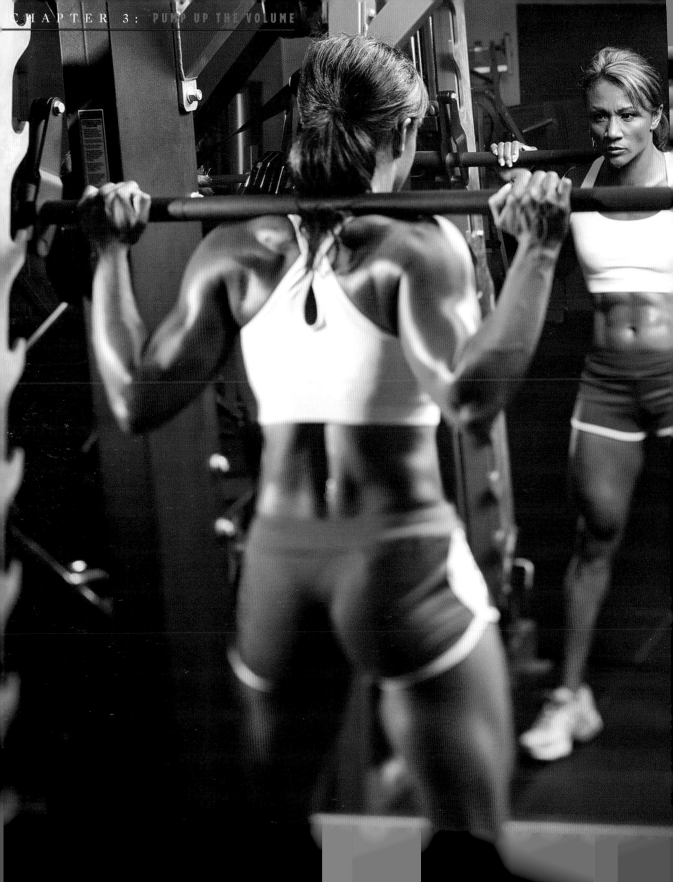

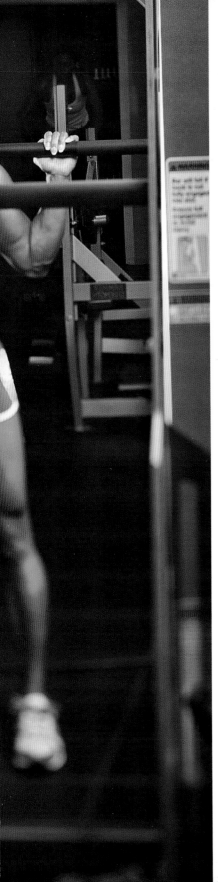

Rest-Pause Sets

WHAT IT IS: A set in which you reach failure, then rest a short period and continue to failure using the same weight. A typical set consists of 1–3 rest-pauses.

WHY DO IT: Like dropsets, rest-pauses allow you to take a set of a given exercise past the point of muscle failure, which can promote gains in muscle size, strength, and shape. But in this case, the short rest period allows you to stick with the same weight instead of going lighter. As a result, what was once a set of 10 reps with 100 pounds becomes a set of 15–20 reps with 100 pounds, so more total work is performed.

HOW TO DO IT: Performing a rest-pause set is very straightforward: Using the weight you'd normally lift for a given exercise, go to failure, rest 15 seconds, then rep to failure again with the same weight. Repeat 1–2 more times. The number of reps you can perform will decrease significantly with each rest-pause set, so don't expect to fail at 10 reps, rest 15 seconds, then get another 10. Chances are you'll be able to get only 3–5 more reps, tops. And if you do another rest-pause set, you'll get even fewer. One way to avoid a big dropoff is to stop a couple of reps short of failure on the initial set, which will allow you to get more reps after resting. Either way will work.

Sample Rest-Pause Leg Routine

EXERCISE	SETS	REPS	REST
Smith Machine Squat	4*	8–10	2 min.
Leg Press	3*	10–12	2 min.
Leg Extension	3*	12–15	1–2 min.
Leg Curl	3*	12–15	1–2 min.

Perform 2–3 rest-pauses on the last 1–2 sets.

CHAPTER 4

COUNTDOWN TO ABS

Go from flab to fab with this 12-week progressive diet and exercise plan

Doing hundreds of crunches won't give you the abs you want, but a well-thought-out workout program performed over a sustained period combined with a diet structured with fat loss in mind will. To attain the holy grail of a lean, tight midsection, you must progressively make your abs stronger, burn the flab hiding them, and dial in your diet. This program will help you do that.

The training regimen is broken down into three four-week phases. In Phase 1, you create the basic foundation that lets you proceed to more advanced routines in Phases 2 and 3. And as you progressively work your abdominals harder, you'll refine your diet each week to prepare for the unveiling of those fabulous abs come summertime. The guidelines listed here help you ease into and fine-tune your existing diet, but to really rev up the fat-burning furnace, use this routine in tandem with a balanced diet.

This program is designed to fit into your current workout schedule; just do your regular training and cardio routines as prescribed and swap out your usual ab work for these targeted routines three days a week, resting at least 48 hours between sessions. Now pull out your calendar, mark your unveiling day and start the countdown to fab abs.

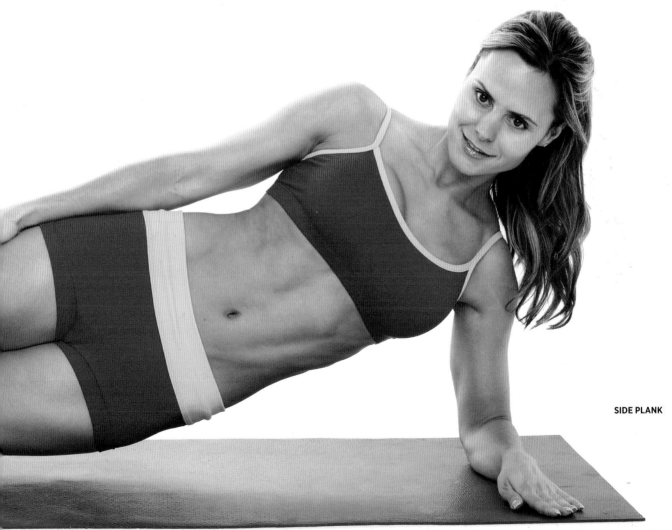

SIDE PLANK

You're 12 weeks out...

MONTH 1: CREATING THE FOUNDATION

This month is about adapting to the exercises that form the foundation of this program. Perform your regular weight-training routine while using the workout below to train your abs three times a week, resting at least 48 hours between sessions. Do cardio at a moderate to high intensity 4–5 days a week for 30 minutes.

EXERCISE	SETS	REPS
Exercise Ball Crunch	2–3	10–15
V-Twist	2–3	10–15 (to each side)
Reverse Crunch	2–3	10–15
Straight-leg Raise	2–3	10–15
Plank	3	25–30 sec.

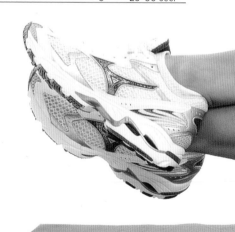

WEEKLY NUTRITION GOALS

12 WEEKS OUT: WRITE IT DOWN

Research shows that people who keep a food journal are more successful at losing and maintaining weight. It simply makes you more accountable: When you write down every morsel you put in your mouth and note how certain foods make you feel or affect your performance mentally and physically, you can easily make adjustments. Continue doing this throughout the program.

11 WEEKS OUT: CARRY WATER

Regular water keeps digestion, nutrient absorption, temperature regulation, and waste elimination running smoothly. Plus, one study found that drinking a half-liter of cold water increased metabolic rate by 30% for more than an hour after drinking.

To calculate your water-intake goals, take your body weight in pounds and divide that number by two. That gives you the minimum number of ounces of water you should drink daily.

10 WEEKS OUT: EAT PROTEIN AT EVERY MEAL

Eating protein makes you feel satisfied, therefore decreasing hunger sensations. If you eat only carbs, you'll crave more; and more carbs can turn into a vicious cycle leading to poor energy and weight gain because of increased calorie intake. Aim to consume 20–30 grams of protein at every meal.

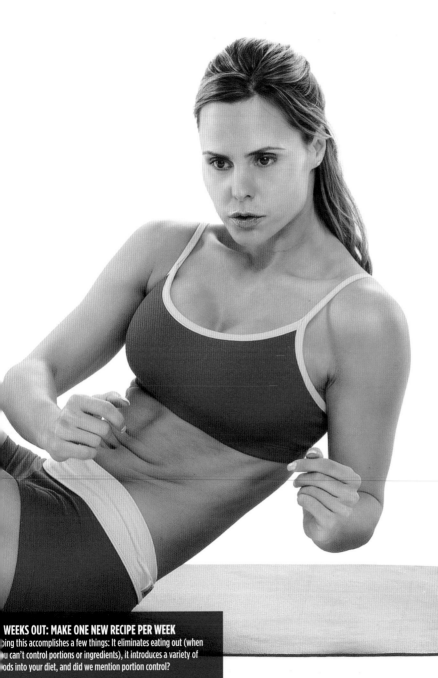

EXERCISE-BALL CRUNCH
TARGETS: UPPER ABS
START: Lie faceup on a large exercise ball with your lower and middle back supported, knees bent, and feet flat on the floor. Cross your arms over your chest. (For increased difficulty, place your hands lightly behind your neck as shown or, to make it even harder, extend your arms overhead.)
MOVEMENT: Raise only your head and shoulders as you contract your abs to move your upper body toward your pelvis. Slowly return to the starting position.

V-TWIST
TARGETS: ALL REGIONS, WITH EMPHASIS ON THE OBLIQUES AND CORE
START: Sit on the floor with your knees slightly bent and hold your arms at 90-degree angles with your hands out in front of you. Lift your feet about 6 inches off the floor. Cross your ankles and lean back about 45 degrees while balancing on your glutes.
MOVEMENT: Pull your belly button toward your lower back, then rotate your torso to the left so your right shoulder points toward your knees. Twist to the right and repeat; continue twisting until you've done 10 reps to each side, or 20 total.

REVERSE CRUNCH
TARGETS: LOWER ABS
START: Lie faceup on the floor, feet up and thighs perpendicular to the floor. Place your arms down by your sides, palms on the floor.
MOVEMENT: Using your lower abs, bring your knees to your chest. Return slowly to the starting position and repeat.

PLANK
TARGETS: CORE
START: Lie facedown on the floor and prop yourself up on your forearms with your elbows bent 90 degrees. Extend your legs and flex your feet so your toes touch the floor.
MOVEMENT: Keeping your abs pulled in tight and your back flat, lift your hips so your body weight is supported by your forearms and toes. Hold this position for up to 30 seconds. Maintain a tight low back and squeeze your glutes to prevent your body from sagging in the middle.

STRAIGHT-LEG RAISE
TARGETS: LOWER ABS
START: Lie faceup on a bench with your glutes at its edge. Extend your legs, keeping them parallel to the floor. Place your hands next to your head and grasp the sides of the bench, or near your hips.
MOVEMENT: Keeping your legs as straight as possible, raise them slowly until you're in a jackknife position. Your head and shoulders shouldn't move—make sure your abs do all the work. Unfold your body slowly and under control, lowering your legs back to the start position. Don't allow your feet to drop below the plane of the bench.

WEEKS OUT: MAKE ONE NEW RECIPE PER WEEK
ing this accomplishes a few things: It eliminates eating out (when u can't control portions or ingredients), it introduces a variety of ods into your diet, and did we mention portion control?

WEIGHTED SINGLE-LEG PLANK

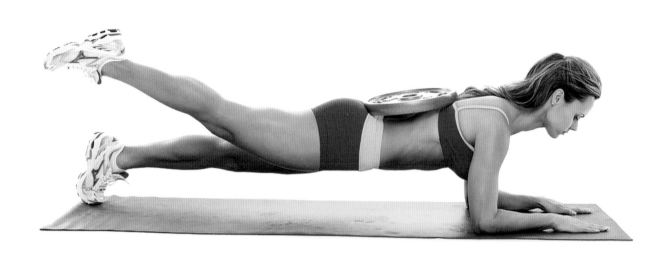

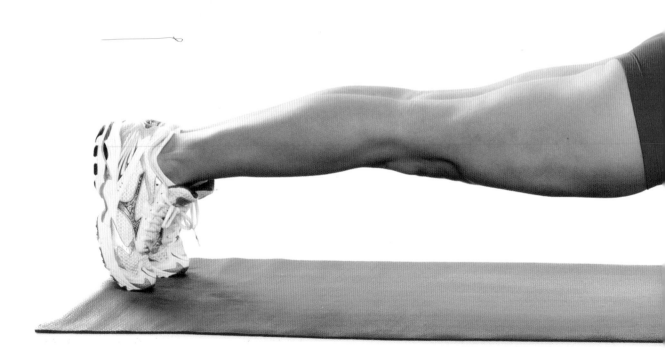

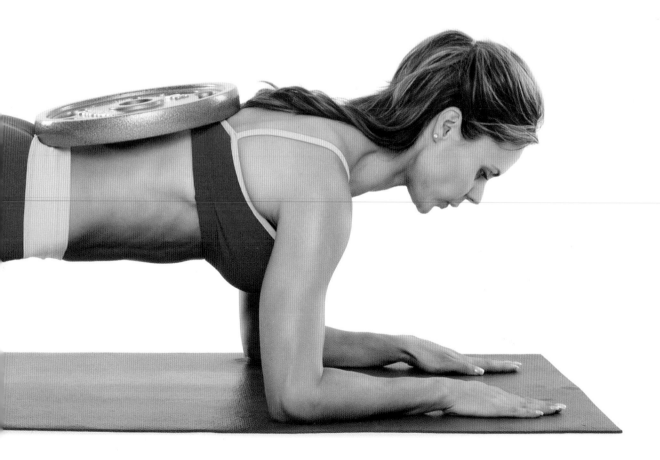

You're 8 weeks away...

MONTH 2: MAKING PROGRESS AND MUSCLE DEFINITION

Time to build some muscle. This month, add weight to the exercises from Month 1. Just like last month, do the program below in the order listed three days a week, resting at least 48 hours between workouts. In addition, perform your regular weight-training routine and increase your cardio to 45 minutes per session 4–5 days a week.

EXERCISE	SETS	REPS
Exercise-ball Crunch		
With Medicine Ball	3	12
Weighted V-Twist	2	10
		(each side)
Hip Thrust with		
Medicine Ball	3	10
Weighted Plank	3	25–30 sec.

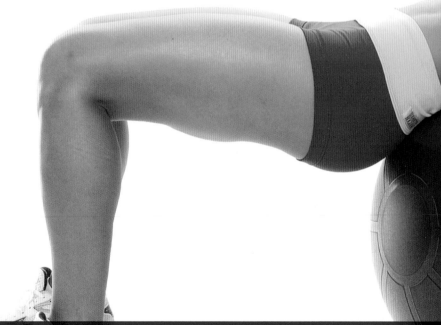

WEEKLY NUTRITION GOALS
8 WEEKS OUT: LOAD UP ON FRUITS AND VEGETABLES
Consider the colors of your fruits and vegetables as your map to beneficial phytochemicals and antioxidants. Each color represents different phytochemicals that work in different parts of your body's cells. Consuming a rainbow of foods during the day helps fight off the cell damage that intense exercise can provoke.

7 WEEKS OUT: FORGET LATE-NIGHT MUNCHIES
Avoid eating three hours before bed. However, if you must, eat protein like low-fat cottage cheese, a part-skim mozzarella cheese stick, or a boiled egg. Do not eat carbs during this three-hour period, since any food intake is more easily stored as fat when you're asleep.

6 WEEKS OUT: AVOID DRINKING YOUR CALORIES
Consider this: Drinking a 10-ounce glass of fruit juice each day can add 51,100 calories in a year, or nearly 15 pounds. Tired of water? Drink green tea or coffee; both benefit your health and training without calories. Green tea contains antioxidants and can help burn fat. Coffee has been shown to improve performance in the gym when consumed before training.

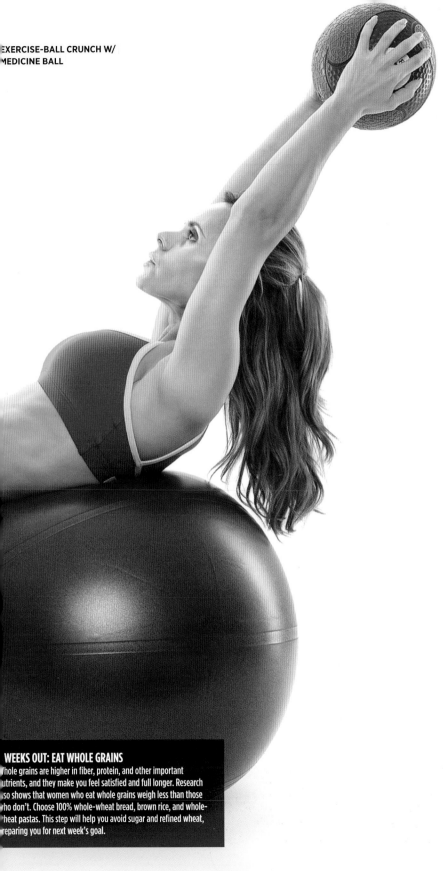

EXERCISE-BALL CRUNCH W/
MEDICINE BALL

WEIGHTED V-TWIST

TARGETS: ALL REGIONS, WITH EMPHASIS ON THE OBLIQUES AND CORE

START: Sit on the floor with your legs extended but slightly bent. Hold a medicine ball with both hands in front of your abdominals and bend your arms slightly. Cross your ankles and lean your upper body back about 45 degrees. Elevate your feet about six inches off the floor.

MOVEMENT: Twist your torso to one side until the ball touches the floor. Smoothly return to center, then repeat the motion to the other side. Keep your abs tight throughout the exercise. Do 10 reps to each side.

EXERCISE-BALL CRUNCH WITH MEDICINE BALL

TARGETS: UPPER ABS

START: Lie faceup on a large exercise ball with your lower and middle back supported, knees bent, and feet flat on the floor. Hold a medicine ball securely overhead at arm's length.

MOVEMENT: Raise your head and shoulders as you crunch your ribcage toward your pelvis. Keep your arms straight so that the medicine ball is overhead. Contract your abs at the top of the movement for a one-count.

HIP THRUST WITH MEDICINE BALL

TARGETS: LOWER ABS

START: Lie faceup on the floor with your arms at your sides, palms down, holding a medicine ball securely between your knees. Lift your legs until your thighs are perpendicular to the floor.

MOVEMENT: Use your abs to lift your hips. At first this will be only a few inches off the floor; the stronger you get, the higher you'll be able to lift.

WEIGHTED PLANK

TARGETS: CORE

START: Lie facedown on the floor with a weight plate balanced on your lower back. Prop yourself up onto your forearms with your elbows bent 90 degrees. Extend your legs and flex your feet so your toes touch the floor.

MOVEMENT: Keeping your abs pulled in tight and your back flat, lift your hips so your forearms and toes support your body weight. Hold for 30 seconds.

WEEKS OUT: EAT WHOLE GRAINS
Whole grains are higher in fiber, protein, and other important nutrients, and they make you feel satisfied and full longer. Research also shows that women who eat whole grains weigh less than those who don't. Choose 100% whole-wheat bread, brown rice, and whole-wheat pastas. This step will help you avoid sugar and refined wheat, preparing you for next week's goal.

BOAT SIT

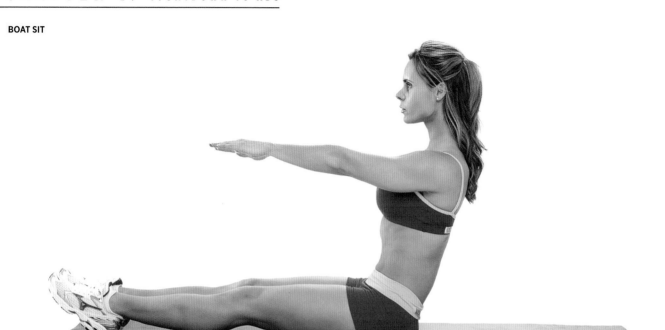

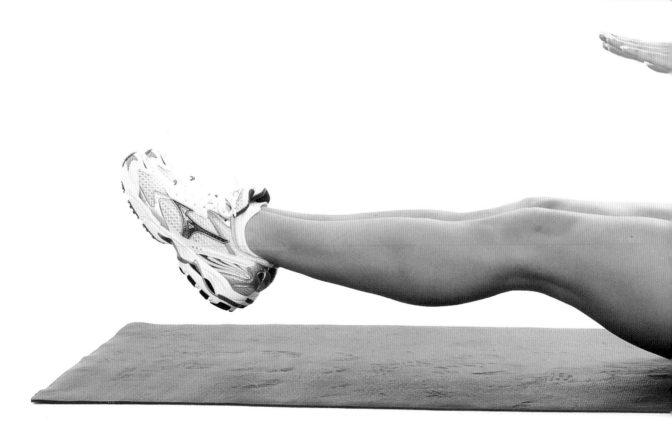

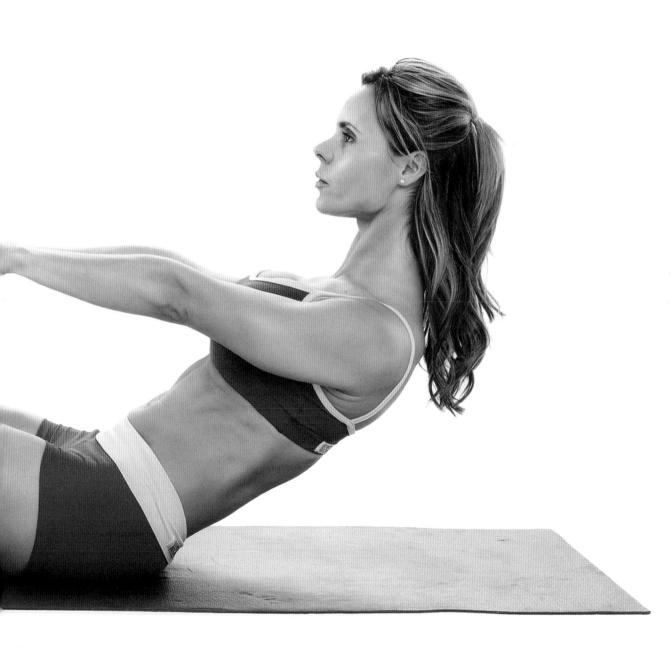

Only 4 more weeks!

MONTH 3: THE FINAL STRETCH

Welcome to the last four weeks of your fab ab journey. This month's goal is to build muscle endurance. Just as you did in Months 1 and 2, perform the program below three days per week, resting at least 48 hours between workouts. In addition, do your regular weight-training routine and increase your cardio to 4–5 days a week, 45–60 minutes per session.

EXERCISE	SETS	REPS
Weighted Single-leg Plank	2	25–30 sec.
Side Plank	2	25–30 sec.
Weighted Plank on Bosu	2	25–30 sec.
Boat Sit	2	25–30 sec.

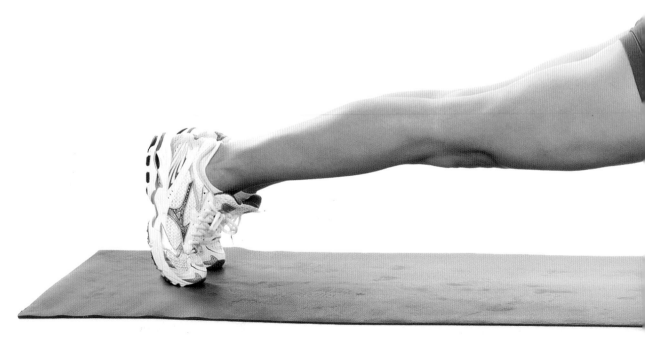

...IGHTED
...NGLE-LEG PLANK
...RGETS: CORE
...RT: Lie facedown on ...floor with a weight ...e balanced on your ...r back. Prop yourself ...onto your forearms ...h your elbows bent 90 ...rees. Extend your legs ...l flex your feet so your ...s touch the floor.
...RIATION: Keeping ...r abs pulled in tight ...l your back flat, lift ...r hips so your fore-...s and toes support ...r body weight. Main-...a tight low back and ...eeze your glutes to ...vent your body from ...ging in the middle. Lift ...e foot off the ground ...2 inches while keeping ...r back flat. Hold this ...ition as long as you ..., working your way up ...0 seconds. Lower and ...eat on the other foot.

SIDE PLANK
TARGETS: CORE
START: Lie on your left side with your legs extended. Prop yourself up on your left elbow, which should be directly below your shoulder.
MOVEMENT: Keeping your left elbow and left foot in contact with the floor, raise your hips as high as possible without rolling forward or back. Keep your body in a straight line and your abs tight. Hold this position as long as you can, working up to 20 seconds. Slowly lower your hips to return to the starting position, and repeat for reps. Switch sides and repeat.

WEIGHTED PLANK ON BOSU
TARGETS: CORE
START: Kneel on all fours with your arms on the flat side of a Bosu and a weight plate balanced on your back. Position your elbows under your shoulders and extend your forearms and hands forward. Extend your legs and flex your feet so your toes touch the floor. You may need a training partner to place the plate.
MOVEMENT: Keeping your abs pulled in tight and your back flat, lift your hips so your fore-arms and toes support your body weight. Hold this position for up to 30 seconds. Maintain a tight lower back and squeeze your glutes to prevent your body from sagging in the middle.

As a warmup, perform this exercise without the plate to get used to the instability of the Bosu.

BOAT SIT
TARGETS: CORE
START: Sit on the floor with your legs extended, abs tight, and back straight. Extend your arms in front of you so they're parallel to the floor.
MOVEMENT: Lean back 45 degrees, then lift your feet off the floor about 6 inches. Hold for as long as possible while maintaining good form; work up to 30 seconds.

WEEKLY NUTRITION GOALS

4 WEEKS OUT: EAT "CLEAN"
Start eating clean, which means you need to eat more fresh fruits and vegetables, whole grains, low-fat dairy, nuts, seeds, and lean meats and fish. Minimize the intake of foods with preservatives, artificial ingredients, chemically altered fats, and high sodium.

3 WEEKS OUT: SUBTRACT ADDED SUGAR
Consider that the average American consumes 20 teaspoons of added sugar daily—in the forms of corn syrup, glucose, and table sugar added into processed foods—and that adds about 320 calories per day. Cutting these unwanted calories can help you lose the fat that seems to be holding onto your midsection.

2 WEEKS OUT: REVISIT YOUR JOURNAL
Two weeks to your goal, how's your diet? Look over your food journal entries. Have you been eating enough protein? How's your vegetable intake? Can you crank each up a notch? Identify the areas in which you might have been a bit lax and renew your commitment.

1 WEEK OUT: ELIMINATE SALT
At this point, you have only seven days until it's time to reveal your abs at the pool, beach, or gym. So if you've been using frozen meals for portion control, canned vegetables to get your five-a-day, or deli meat for your protein fix, say no to them this week because they contain higher levels of sodium than fresh foods. Too much of this mineral can promote water retention and bloating—two things that can hide your hard-earned ab definition. Look at your journal to identify the sneaky ways salt gets in your diet, and cut it back. It may mean breaking up with your saltshaker.

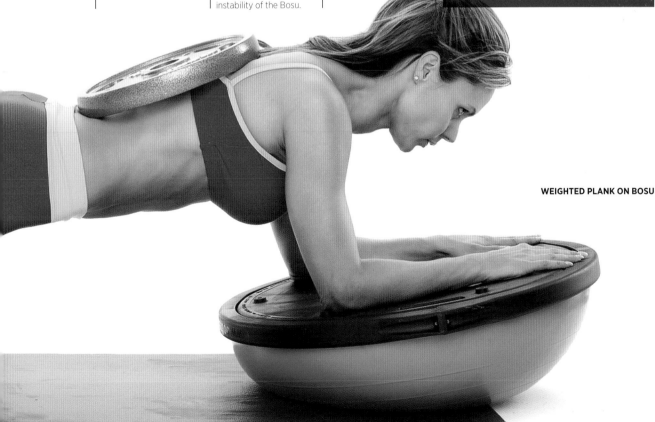

WEIGHTED PLANK ON BOSU

CHAPTER 5

GOT GLUTES?

Use these 10 exercises to whip your backside into shape

Buns. Booty. Assets. Badonkadonk. No matter what you call your backside, you want it to be as high, tight, round, and firm as possible. Six-pack abs are awesome—but you know the truest test of sex appeal comes from a sleek derrière.

Getting it is another matter, since this is the spot where women tend to hold the most body fat for the longest time. Thankfully, Kim Oddo, trainer to the fitness stars, and IFBB figure pro (and mother of three) Cheryl Brown are here to show you how to kick your own ass into the shape you want with 10 moves specifically designed to improve your bottom line.

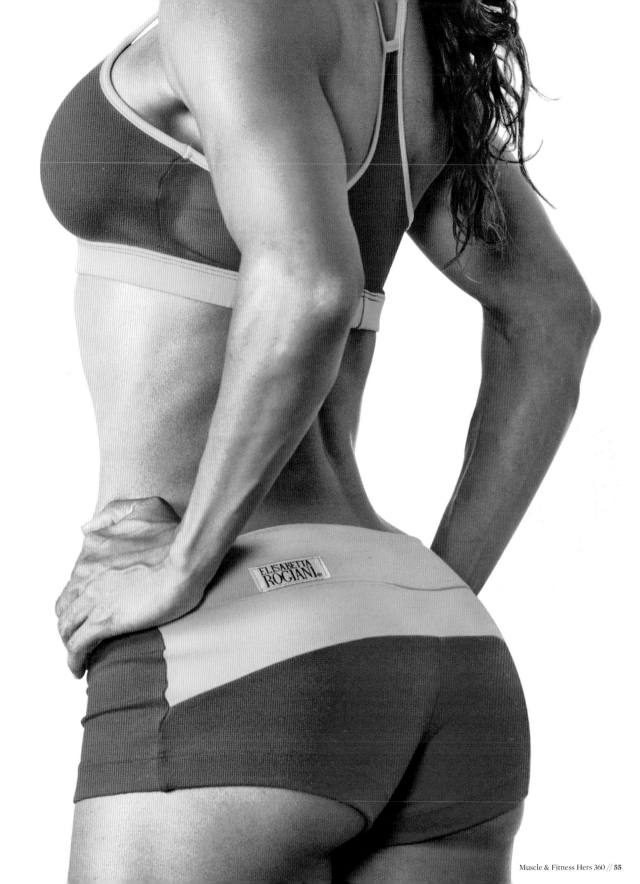

Unilateral Stiff-Leg Deadlift

DEGREE OF DIFFICULTY: * (THREE STARS)**

Overview: The key to making this exercise target the glutes instead of the hamstrings is the stretch.

Get Ready: With your feet close together, hold a dumbbell in your right hand with an overhand grip and extend your arm. Keep your head up and a tight arch in the small of your back.

Go: Bending your right knee slightly and keeping your left leg straight and locked, hinge at the hips to lower your torso toward the floor, using the weight as a counterbalance as your left leg comes up in a straight line behind you. With contracted abs, squeeze your right glute and hamstring as you pull your torso back to vertical. Repeat for reps before switching legs.

ODDO'S TIP:
"Girls tend to be more flexible than guys, so do these standing on a box for a greater range of motion."

STRAIGHT-SET WORKOUT

Perform these moves in a traditional three-set format, resting 60 to 90 seconds between each set. Complete all sets for one exercise before moving on to the next.

EXERCISE	SETS/REPS
Single-leg Smith Machine Box Squat (per leg)	3/18, 15, 15
Wide-stance Leg Press	3/18, 15, 15
Leg Press Kickback	3/18, 15, 15
Single-leg Stability Ball Glute Cable Kickback (per leg)	3/18, 15, 15
Unilateral Stiff-leg Deadlift (per leg)	3/20

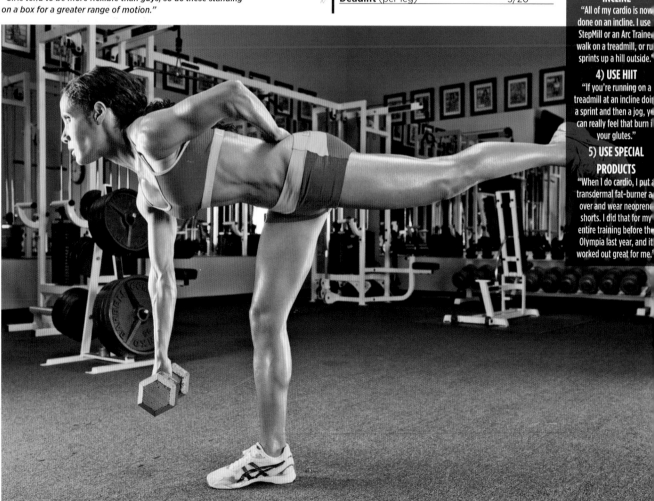

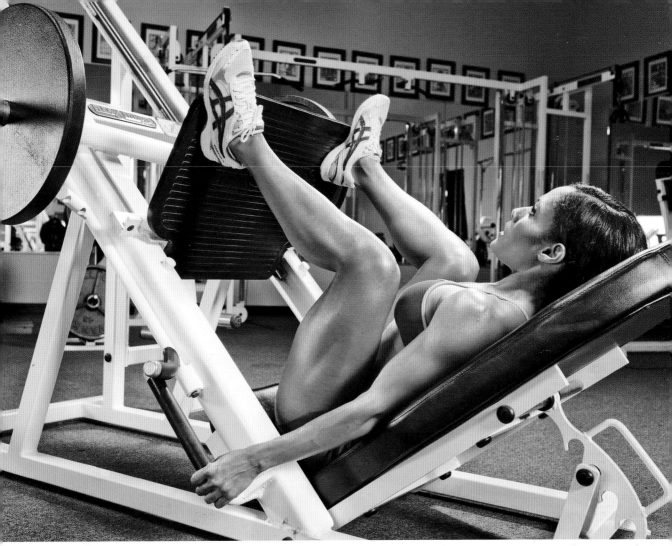

Wide-Stance Leg Press

DEGREE OF DIFFICULTY: *****

Overview: The wide stance transfers the action from the quads to the glutes and hamstrings.

Get Ready: Lying back in a 45-degree leg press machine, place your feet high on the platform so only your heels are resting on it the top outside corners, toes pointed out at 45-degree angles.

Go: Unhinge the weight, then bend your knees to bring the platform toward your chest. Pause for one count, then squeeze your glutes and hamstrings to press the weight back up.

●DO'S TIP:
Make sure the small of your back stays flush against e pad. It's very easy for your glutes to come up, but at can create lower-back injuries."

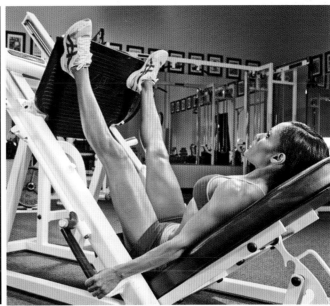

Lateral Step-Up with Kickback

DEGREE OF DIFFICULTY: ***

Overview: This exercise works both the adductors and abductors, but the kickback targets the glutes. To add difficulty, use ankle weights.

Get Ready: Stand to the left side of an aerobic step or box.

Go: Step sideways onto the box with your right leg only, then contract your abs and squeeze your left glute as you bring your straight left leg behind you in a kickback motion. Hold for one count, then release the glute and step carefully off the box with your left leg, followed by your right. Repeat for reps, then switch sides.

ODDO'S TIP:

"Be careful not to spring up. You don't want to get a bounce motion in there. You're isolating the step up and the squeeze-hold to make sure you're not using your calves."

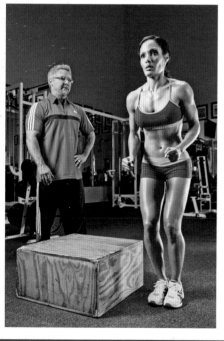

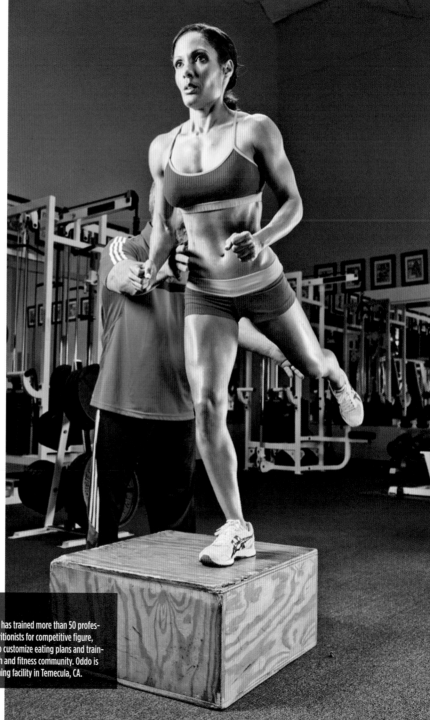

ABOUT KIM ODDO

During his 20 years of experience in the health and fitness industry, Oddo has trained more than 50 professional athletes and established himself as one of the top trainers and nutritionists for competitive figure, bikini, and fitness athletes in the world. His keen understanding of how to customize eating plans and training programs for each client has given him a special standing in the health and fitness community. Oddo is the owner and operator of Body By O, a 3,000-square-foot personal-training facility in Temecula, CA.

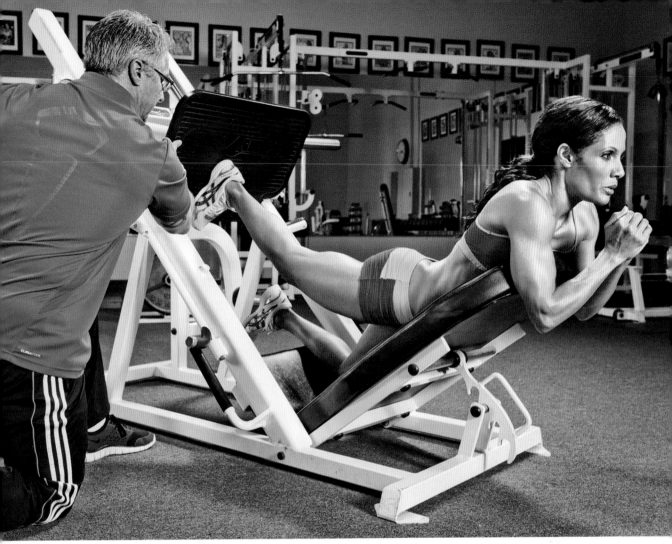

Leg Press
Kickback

DEGREE OF DIFFICULTY: ****

Overview: If your gym doesn't have a dedicated Butt Blaster machine, use this instead—it uses the same range of motion and targets the middle portion and upper crest of the glutes.

Get Ready: Turn yourself around in a 45-degree leg press machine so your stomach and elbows are resting on the back pad, knees on the seat. Put one foot in the middle of the platform.

Go: Unhinge the weight, then press your foot back at a 45-degree angle by straightening your leg, squeezing the glutes at the top. Return halfway to the starting position, then repeat for reps.

ODDO'S TIP:
"Don't arch your back. Make sure your foot is square so your toes are pointing straight down, and don't use a weight that's too heavy."

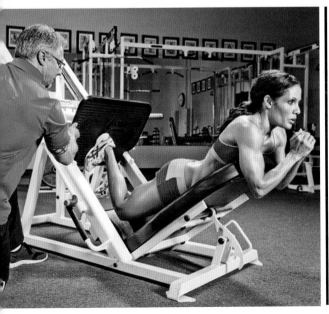

Split Squat

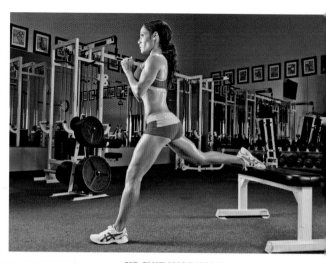

DEGREE OF DIFFICULTY: ★★★★

Overview: This exercise works both glutes at the same time—one gets stretched while the other is contracted. To add difficulty, use a stability ball instead of a bench.

Get Ready: Stand a few feet in front of a bench. Carefully extend one foot back to place it on top of the bench with the sole of your shoe almost parallel to the floor.

Go: Bend your front leg to lower your torso straight down toward the ground, making sure your knee stays behind your toes, until your thigh is about parallel to the ground and your back knee is within a foot of the floor. Press through the heel of your front leg and squeeze your glute as you rise straight back up.

ODDO'S TIP:

"Make sure the movement goes straight down, not forward."

CIRCUIT WORKOUT

Perform one set of each exercise followed by one set of the next exercise until you have completed all exercises. Run through this circuit three times, resting 30 seconds between each round.

EXERCISE	SETS/REPS (PER CIRCUIT)
Lateral Step-up with Kickback (per leg)	3/25, 20, 18
Split Squat (per leg)	3/25, 20, 18
Side Band Walking (per leg)	3/30, 25, 20
Medicine Ball Hip Thrust	3/30
Wall Squat with Stability Ball	3/25, 20, 18

Single-Leg Smith Machine Box Squat

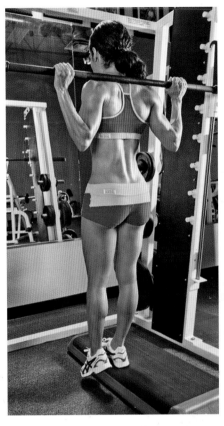

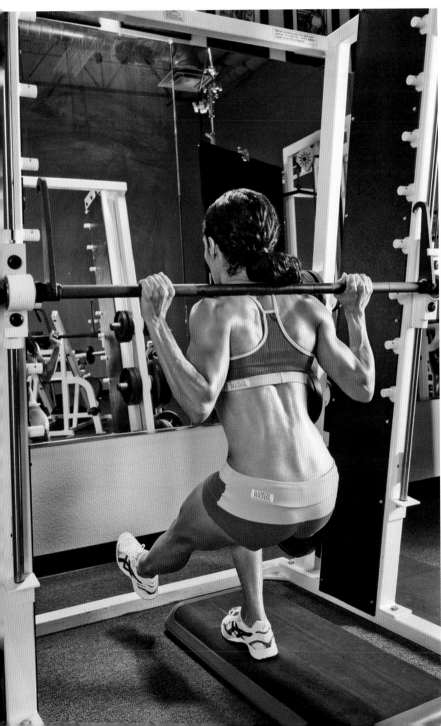

DEGREE OF DIFFICULTY: *****

Overview: Do this near the beginning of your workout, when your legs are fresh and you can really focus on the glutes.

Get Ready: Set up an aerobic step inside a Smith machine and, resting the bar across your upper traps, stand with one foot on the platform and the other hanging straight down. Unrack the bar and extend your free leg forward at about a 45-degree angle while keeping the other foot planted on the platform.

Go: Keeping your back flat, descend until your working quad is just past parallel to the floor. Press up through the heel, shifting your hips forward and squeezing your glutes to return to standing.

ODDO'S TIP:
"Make sure you don't go too far down past parallel; anything more will put stress on the patella. Make sure not to bounce the motion."

Single-Leg Stability-Ball Glute Cable Kickback

DEGREE OF DIFFICULTY: **

Overview: Working one leg at a time helps erase muscle imbalances; try using different ranges of motion to see what works best for you.

Get Ready: Attach an ankle collar to a cable pulley at the lowest setting. Wrap the strap around one ankle, then step about three feet away from the pole. Lie facedown on a stability ball so your stomach and upper thighs rest on it, then place the toes of your nonworking foot on the floor behind you and your hands shoulder-width apart on the floor in front of you.

Go: Lock your ankle and, keeping your knee slightly bent, curl your heel toward the ceiling, keeping your hips pressed into the ball. Hold for one count and squeeze your glute, then slowly lower your toe back to the floor.

ODDO'S TIP:
"Keep your head and neck parallel with the floor throughout the exercise."

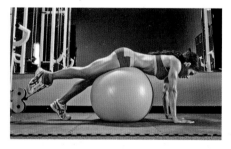

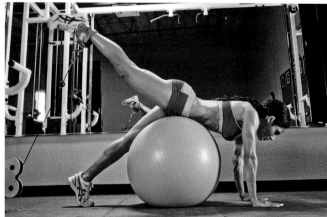

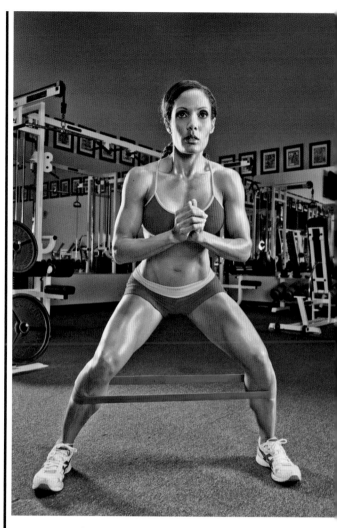

Side Band Walking

DEGREE OF DIFFICULTY: ***

Overview: This exercise effectively targets the glute-ham tie-in, where most women tend to carry body fat.

Get Ready: Tie a resistance band just below your knees, and descend into a quarter-squat position, feet slightly more than shoulder-width apart to put tension on the band.

Go: Keeping your abs tight and staying in the quarter-squat, step to the right with your right leg first, then your left, keeping tension on the band throughout. Repeat for reps, then switch sides to lead with your left leg.

ODDO'S TIP:
"I really like this one because it hits an area in your glutes that's really hard to get to."

Medicine-Ball Hip Thrust

DEGREE OF DIFFICULTY: ****

Overview: By rolling the medicine ball closer to or farther away from your glutes, you will feel this exercise in different areas of your glutes. Find the place that allows you to feel it most in the lower-middle portion of your glutes. For added resistance, place a dumbbell or weight plate on your pelvis.

Get Ready: Lie on your back on the floor with your knees bent and your heels on a small medicine ball.

Go: Contract your abs, then squeeze your glutes and hamstrings to thrust your hips upward. Hold for a count, then lower yourself three-quarters of the way back to the floor, keeping your abs contracted, and repeat.

ODDO'S TIP:
"Keep your head on the floor. Doing this with your head up is a good way to pinch a nerve in your neck."

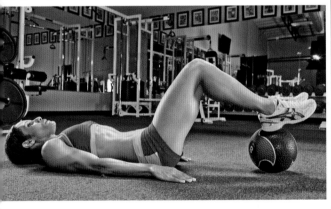

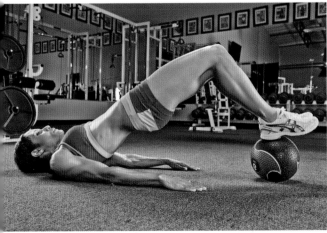

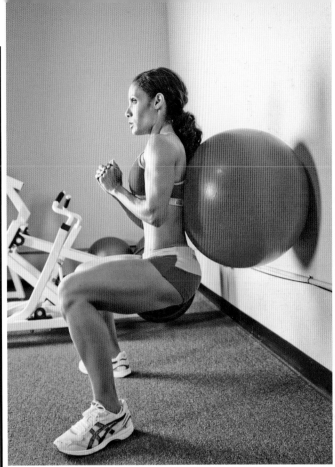

Wall Squat with Stability Ball

DEGREE OF DIFFICULTY: ***

Overview: A great isolator for the glutes and hamstrings, this move eliminates danger to the lower back. For added resistance, hold a pair of dumbbells.

Get Ready: Stand facing away from a wall with a stability ball between it and the small of your back. Your feet should be in front of your hips, slightly wider than your shoulders, with toes pointed out at 45-degree angles.

Go: Keeping your feet flat on the floor, squat down so the ball rolls up your back, until your quads are just past parallel to the floor. Hold for a count, then lift just your toes into the air to push through your heels as you rise back to the starting position, rotating your glutes and hams inward. Lower your toes back to the floor before starting the next rep.

ODDO'S TIP:
"This is not your typical squatting motion. I hate to use this analogy, but it's kind of like holding and squeezing a pencil [between your glutes]."

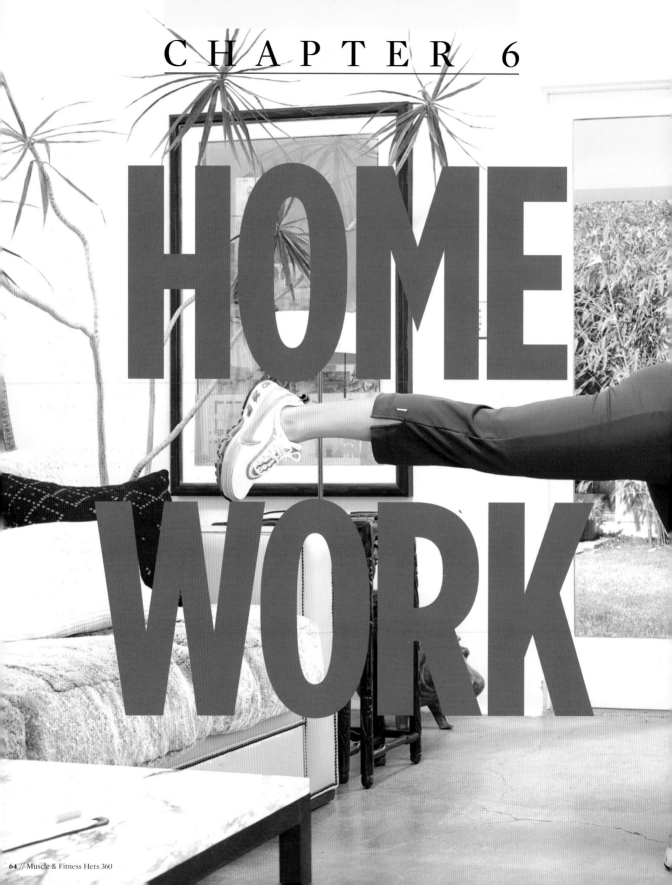

CHAPTER 6

HOME WORK

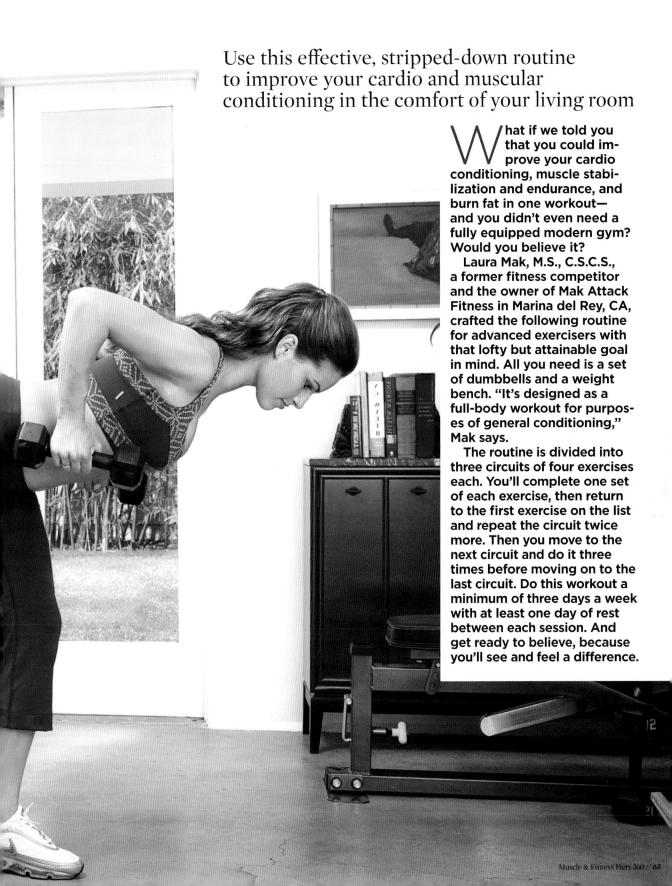

Use this effective, stripped-down routine to improve your cardio and muscular conditioning in the comfort of your living room

What if we told you that you could improve your cardio conditioning, muscle stabilization and endurance, and burn fat in one workout—and you didn't even need a fully equipped modern gym? Would you believe it?

Laura Mak, M.S., C.S.C.S., a former fitness competitor and the owner of Mak Attack Fitness in Marina del Rey, CA, crafted the following routine for advanced exercisers with that lofty but attainable goal in mind. All you need is a set of dumbbells and a weight bench. "It's designed as a full-body workout for purposes of general conditioning," Mak says.

The routine is divided into three circuits of four exercises each. You'll complete one set of each exercise, then return to the first exercise on the list and repeat the circuit twice more. Then you move to the next circuit and do it three times before moving on to the last circuit. Do this workout a minimum of three days a week with at least one day of rest between each session. And get ready to believe, because you'll see and feel a difference.

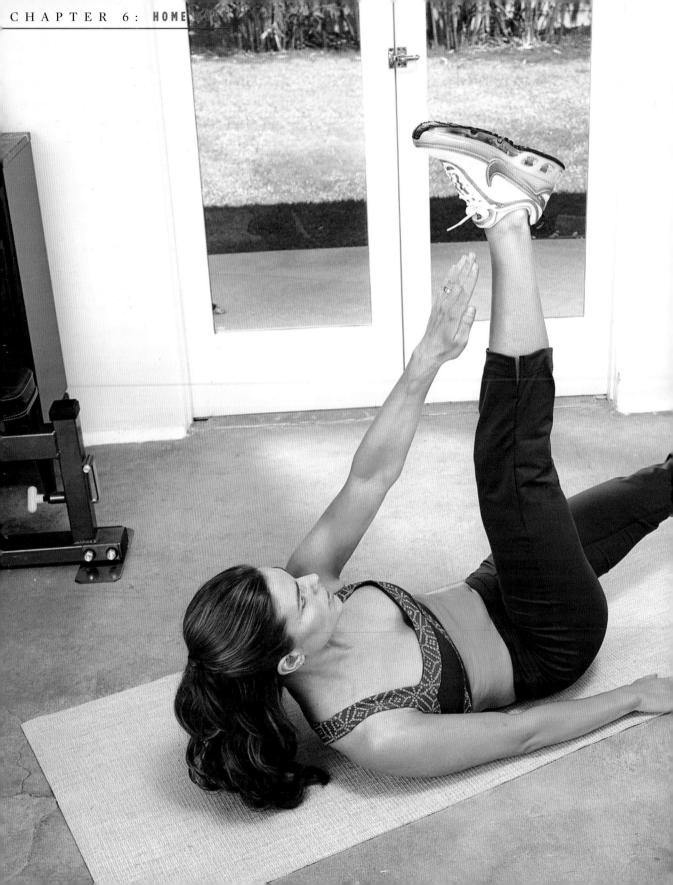

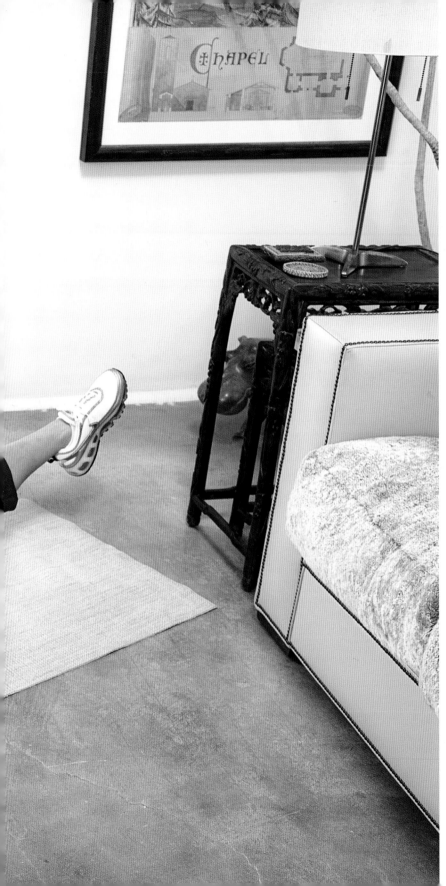

The Routine

Warm up for five minutes any way you like—using cardio equipment, jumping rope, or doing jumping jacks. Whatever you choose, make sure you perform continuous and rhythmic movements using large muscle groups (legs, chest, or back). Then start Circuit 1. Do one set of each exercise on the list, then start again with the first exercise. Repeat this sequence twice more so that you complete the circuit three times, having done three sets of each exercise listed before beginning the next circuit.

Perform a warmup activity for five minutes.

Circuit 1

EXERCISE	REPS
Pop Squat	10–20
Triple Threat Pushup	10–15 (per setup)
Plié Squat Hold with Hammer Curl	15–20
Single Straight-leg Crunch	50

Perform three times, then start Circuit 2.

Circuit 2

EXERCISE	REPS
Split Squat Jump	20 total
Bent-arm Lateral Raise to Overhead Dumbbell Press	10
Overhead Dumbbell Triceps Extension on One Leg	12
Straight-leg Crossover Crunch	60

Perform three times, then start Circuit 3.

Circuit 3

EXERCISE	REPS
Lateral Jump	10
One-leg Bentover Dumbbell Row	15–20
One-leg Bench Dip	24
Bicycle Crunch	30

Perform a cooldown activity for 5–10 minutes.

STRAIGHT-LEG CROSSOVER CRUNCH
TARGETS: Upper and Lower Abs, Obliques
START: Lie faceup on the floor with your right leg perpendicular to your body and your left leg just off the floor. Place your right hand lightly to the side.
MOVEMENT: Crunch up as you reach your left hand toward the outside of your right ankle. Reverse the motion to return to the start. Repeat for reps, then switch sides.

Circuit 1 Exercises

POP SQUAT
TARGETS: Quadriceps, Hamstrings, Glutes
START: Stand erect with your feet together, abs tight, and your arms hanging at your sides (not shown).
MOVEMENT: Bend your knees slightly, then swing your arms toward the ceiling as you jump straight up. Land with your feet turned out about 45 degrees and wider than shoulder-width apart, knees bent about 90 degrees and arms bent in front of you. As soon as you land, immediately rebound into a jump as high as you can and return to the start position with your feet together and arms down. That's one rep.

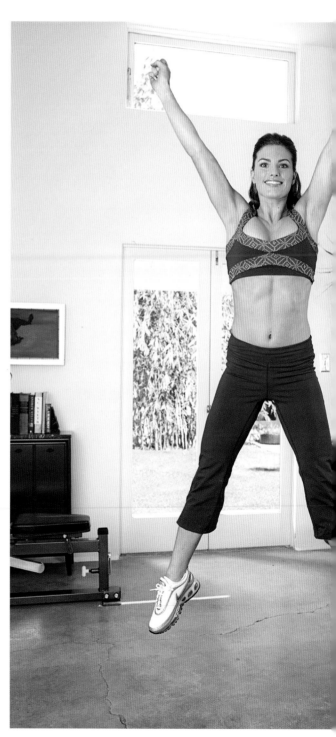

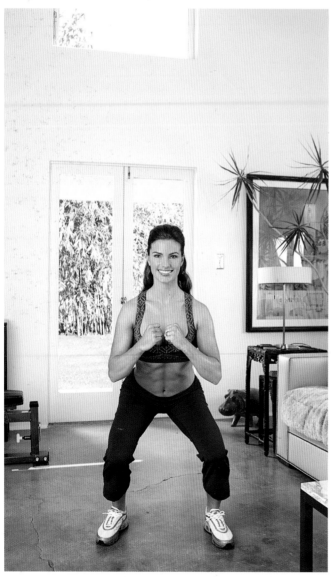

TRIPLE-THREAT PUSHUP

TARGETS: Chest, Shoulders, Triceps

MOVEMENT 1: DECLINE PUSHUP Place your feet up on a bench and space your hands slightly wider than shoulder-width apart on the floor. Keep your abs pulled in tight toward your spine and your body in a straight line from ears to heels. Bend your elbows to lower your chest to the floor. Push back up by contracting your chest and straightening your arms.

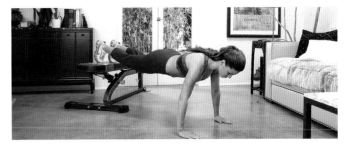

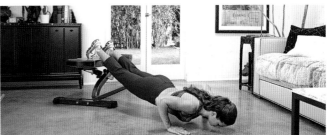

MOVEMENT 2: STANDARD PUSHUP Immediately after your set of decline pushups, move your feet off the bench and onto the floor. Again, keep your body in a straight line from ears to heels with your abs tight. Lower to the floor and push back up.

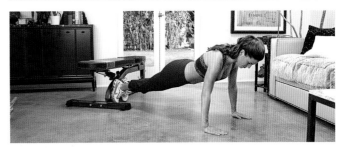

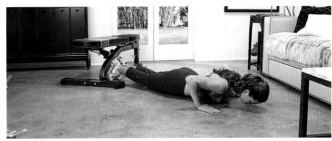

MOVEMENT 3: INCLINE PUSHUP After your standard pushup set, immediately place your hands up on a bench and leave your feet on the floor. Make sure your body remains in a straight line from ears to heels, abs pulled in tight. Lower your chest to the bench and push back up.

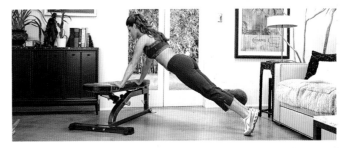

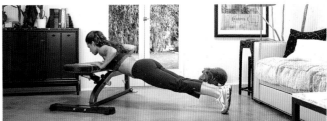

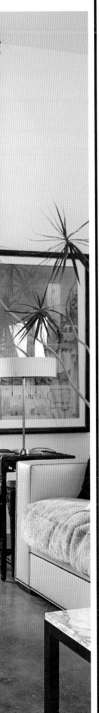

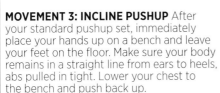

PLIÉ SQUAT HOLD WITH HAMMER CURL

TARGETS: Quadriceps, Hamstrings, Glutes, Biceps

START: Stand with your feet 2–3 feet apart with your toes turned out roughly 45 degrees. Bend your knees about 90 degrees, making sure they don't move past your toes. Hold two dumbbells in front of you, ends together, with your palms facing each other.

MOVEMENT: Lean slightly forward and, with your elbows pressed into your sides, curl the weights toward your shoulders. Reverse the motion to return to the start.

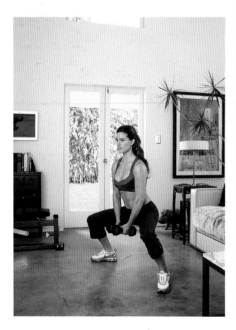

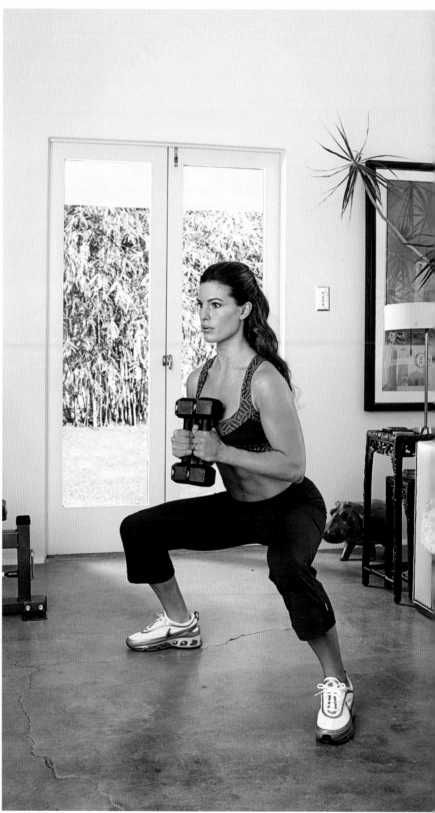

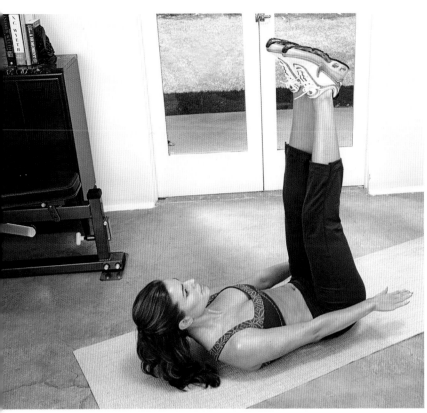

SINGLE STRAIGHT-LEG CRUNCH
TARGET: Abdominals
START: Lie faceup on a bench or the floor and hold your arms slightly elevated next to your sides, extending them toward your feet. Raise your feet so they're directly above your hips and lift your shoulders about 6 inches off the floor.
MOVEMENT: Crunch up with your upper body another 6 inches while simultaneously lowering your left leg so it's 6 inches off the floor. Lower your upper body and bring back your left leg and repeat with your right leg. Perform in a continuous, controlled manner at a moderate speed.

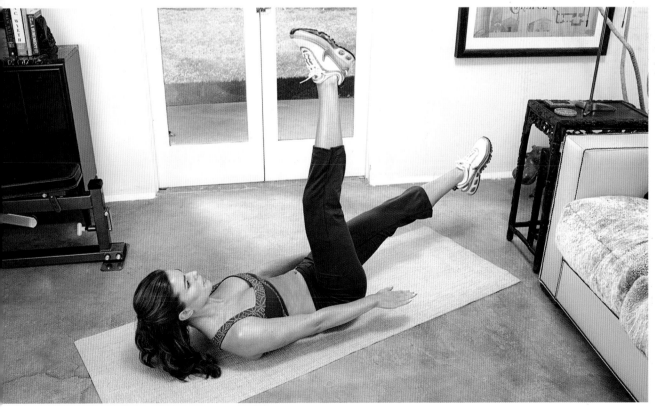

Circuit 2 Exercises

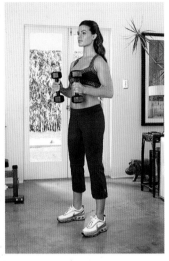
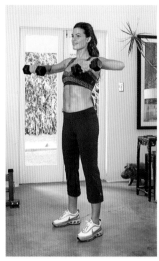
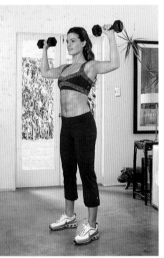
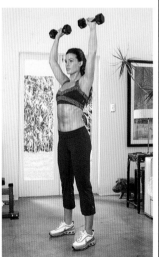

SPLIT SQUAT JUMP

TARGETS: Quadriceps, Hamstrings, Glutes

START: Stand upright in a shoulder-width stance with your hand on your hips. Take a large step forward with your right foot and bend both knees to move into a lunge position.

MOVEMENT: From the bottom of the lunge, jump as high as you can, trying to stay in the air like a basketball player going for a dunk. Before landing, scissor your legs so your left leg is in front. Bend your knees as you land to return to the lunge position. Repeat for reps, alternating sides.

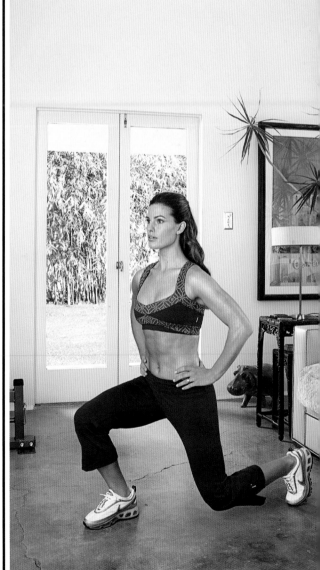

BENT-ARM LATERAL RAISE TO OVERHEAD DUMBBELL PRESS

TARGETS: Deltoids, Triceps

START: Stand upright with your feet shoulder-width apart, abs tight and arms at your sides, grasping a dumbbell in each hand using a neutral grip. Bend your elbows 90 degrees.

MOVEMENT 1: Maintaining the bends in your elbows, raise your arms laterally so they come to shoulder level and are parallel to the floor.

MOVEMENT 2: Rotate your arms, lifting the dumbbells above your elbows so your arms form a goalpost. Press the weights overhead.

MOVEMENT 3: Reverse the movements slowly, returning along the same path to the start position.

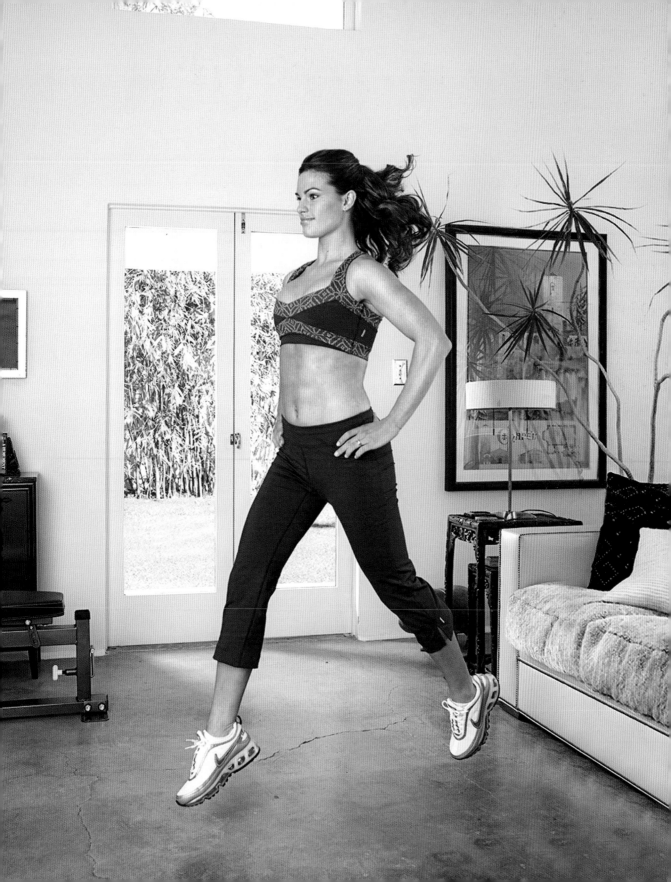

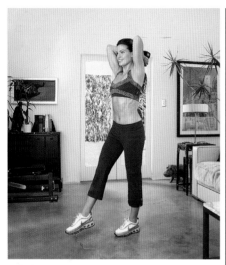

Circuit 3 Exercises

ONE-LEG BENTOVER DUMBBELL ROW
TARGETS: Leg Stabilizers, Abs , Lower Back, Lower Lats
START: Balance on your right foot while keeping your left leg straight, lifting it in front of you at a 45-degree angle. Press two dumbbells overhead (not shown).
MOVEMENT 1: Slowly move your left leg (keeping it extended) behind you until it's parallel to the floor. At the same time, hinge your upper body forward, keeping your arms overhead. Your body should form a straight line from the dumbbells to your left heel.
MOVEMENT 2: Move your arms down so the weights point toward the floor, palms facing in. Then contract your lats to row them up to your hips. Pause, then lower the dumbbells and return them to the overhead position. Then lift your upper body and move your left leg forward to return to the start position. Repeat for reps, then switch sides.

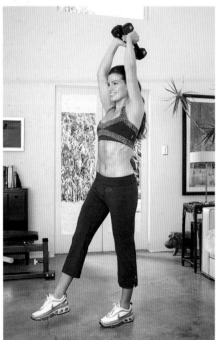

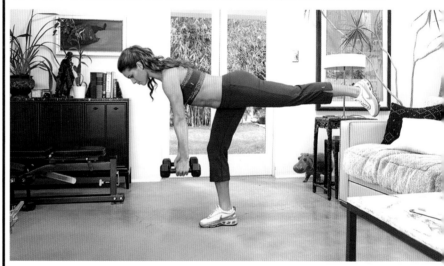

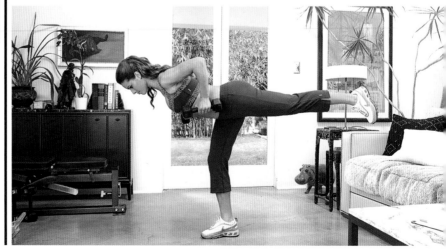

OVERHEAD DUMBBELL TRICEPS EXTENSION ON ONE LEG
TARGETS: Triceps, Balance (stabilizers)
START: Stand on your left foot with your right leg extended in front of you at a 45-degree angle. Don't let your right foot touch the floor. Grasp two dumbbells and press them overhead, holding the ends of the weights together.
MOVEMENT: Keeping your upper arms next to your ears, bend your elbows 90 degrees so the weights move behind your head while maintaining your balance. Repeat for reps, then switch legs. To keep your balance, engage your entire core and keep your shoulder blades down.

LATERAL JUMP

TARGETS: Quadriceps, Hamstrings, Glutes, Calves

START: Stand in a forward lunge position with your right knee bent 90 degrees, reaching your left hand toward the outside of your right ankle, left foot off the floor.

MOVEMENT: Push off with your right foot and jump as high as you can 2–3 feet to the left. Land first on your left foot, bending that knee to 90 degrees and reaching your right hand to the outside of your left ankle. A jump to each side is one rep.

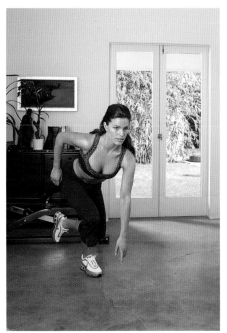
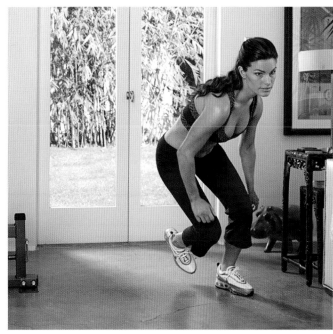

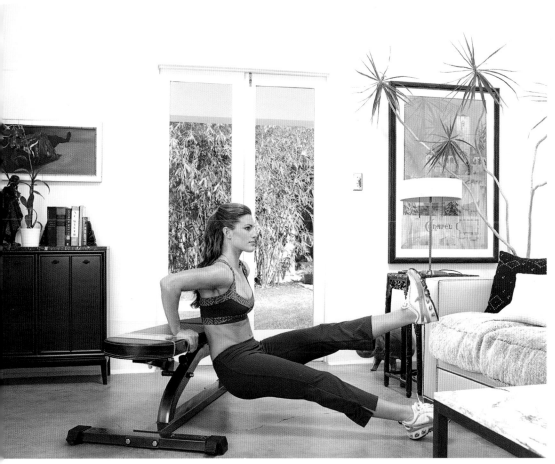

ONE-LEG BENCH DIP

TARGET: Triceps

START: Sit upright along the edge of a bench with your hands next to your hips. Extend your right leg forward, balancing on your heel, and lift your left foot 1–2 feet off the floor. Scoot your hips off the bench, holding your body weight on your hands.

MOVEMENT: Bend your elbows to 90 degrees to lower your body alongside the bench, keeping your left foot up, then push through your hands to straighten your arms. Repeat for reps, then switch sides.

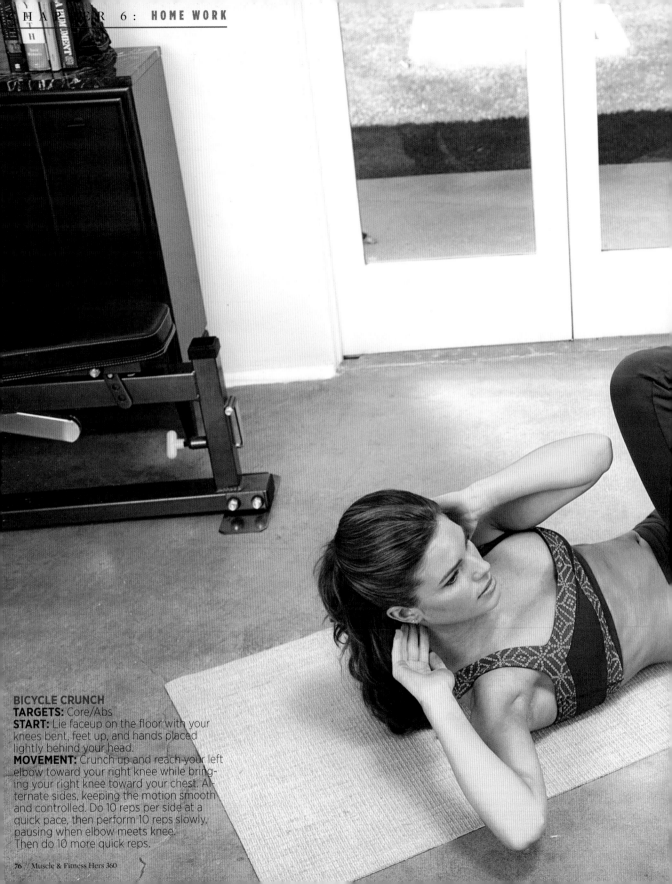

BICYCLE CRUNCH

TARGETS: Core/Abs
START: Lie faceup on the floor with your knees bent, feet up, and hands placed lightly behind your head.
MOVEMENT: Crunch up and reach your left elbow toward your right knee while bringing your right knee toward your chest. Alternate sides, keeping the motion smooth and controlled. Do 10 reps per side at a quick pace, then perform 10 reps slowly, pausing when elbow meets knee. Then do 10 more quick reps.

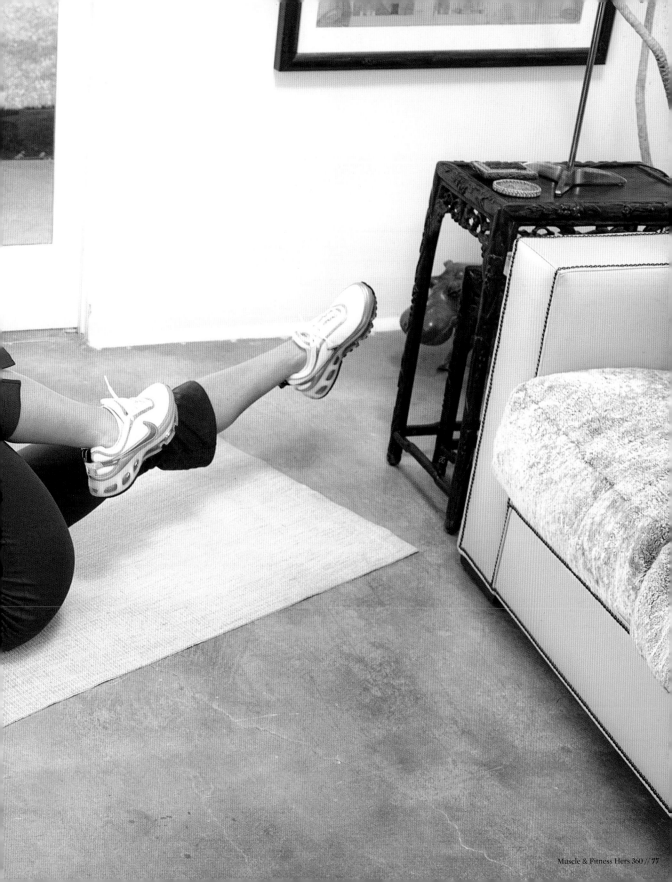

CHAPTER 7

READY, SET, GO!

Crunched for time? No worries. These four 30-minute routines are short on time but long on results.

Sure, it'd be great if everyone had an hour or two every day to commit to fitness. Heck, finding that time could be downright easy if you didn't have to go to work, take care of family obligations, run errands, and sleep. Add the burden of unforeseen circumstances and you may feel as if your quest for a fitter body might just get squeezed out of your schedule altogether. Good news: It doesn't have to be. Don't have 60–90 minutes to spend at the gym? No problem, because we've crammed everything you need into a selection of four potent 30-minute workouts. These ultra-efficient sessions are high on intensity, low on rest, and packed with proven exercises and welcome variety, making them fun and effective.

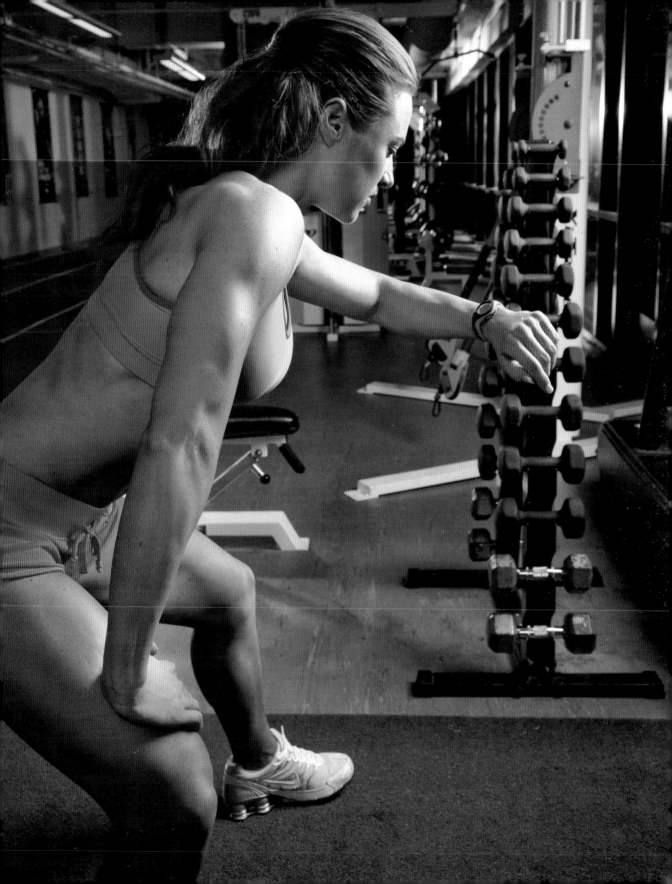

30-Minute Methods

Each of these routines uses several tactics to increase intensity and elicit more benefits in less time. Try them as prescribed and continue experimenting with them in your regular workouts even if you're no longer short on time.

>> SUPERSETS – By completing two exercises back to back with no rest in between, you increase the demand on your muscles and boost the intensity of the training session. The resultant rise in metabolism makes this a must-do technique, especially if time is a factor for you.

>> CONSTANT TENSION – While using free weights is best for getting stronger and leaner in the gym, it's not without its weakness. Some exercises, such as the preacher curl, have "holes" in the movement, where it becomes temporarily easier to execute with free weights. Cables, however, keep tension on the muscle throughout the movement, making certain exercises more effective with them.

>> COMPOUND MOVEMENTS – These multijoint exercises—such as the bench press, squat, and lat pulldown—call on several different muscle groups, meaning you'll break down more muscle fibers than with single-joint moves. Your body's efforts to repair itself burns more calories and you'll come back stronger. Any routine should revolve around these types of exercises.

>> HIGH REPS – High-rep sets not only leave your muscles feeling tight but also provide a higher calorie burn during a workout. High-rep (12 or more) sets also build muscular endurance and athletic performance. Keep your rest periods short (30–45 seconds) for an even greater burn.

>> LOW REPS – Heavier sets (6–8 reps) build strength that's ideal for long-term physique changes and, when paired with shorter rest periods, actually provide a greater increase in your resting metabolic rate for longer after a workout.

>> 100s – While 100 reps in a set seems unfathomable, this type of training taps into every available muscle fiber in a given set. You'll do them here only for calf raises, but 100s training can be applied to nearly any exercise using a weight that's about 20% of your one-rep max. Aim to complete up to 70 reps nonstop, then rest for as many seconds as the number of reps you have remaining. Repeat this pattern until you reach 100 reps. One set per muscle group is plenty, making it perfect when you need to complete as much work in as short a time as possible.

>> DROPSETS – Simply take a muscle to failure, then immediately reduce the weig and continue to failure again. If you have anything left in the tank, you can always drop again. The ideal reduction in weight is 20%–30%. Keep in mind, you should perform dropsets only on the final set of an exercise, to prevent overtraining.

>> VARIETY OF EXERCISES – Incorporat ing unfamiliar movements into your routin places a greater demand on your target muscles. By tapping into underused musc fibers, you enhance your overall muscle quality. Mastering new moves also develo greater mind-muscle coordination.

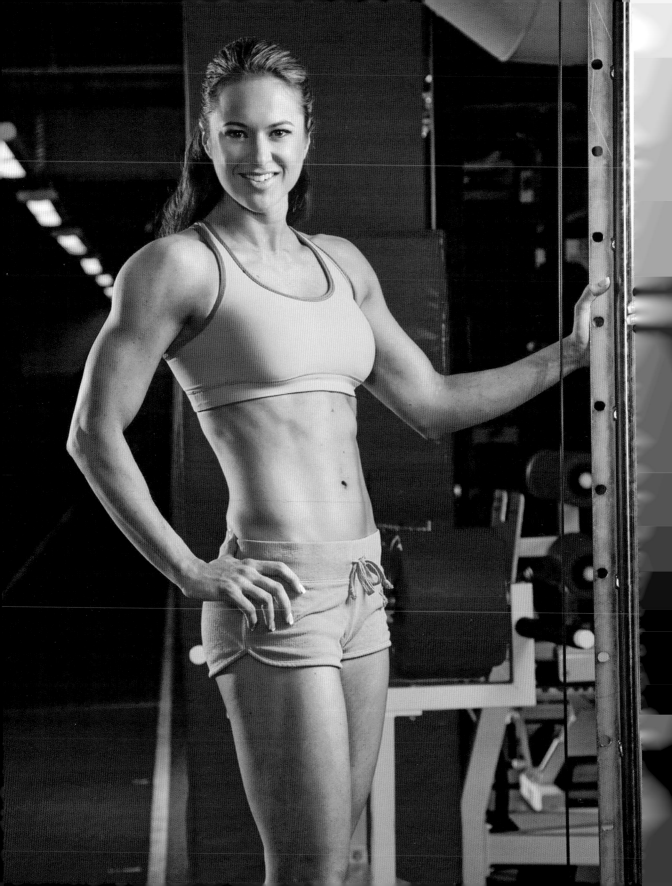

Workout No. 1:
LEGS & SHOULDERS

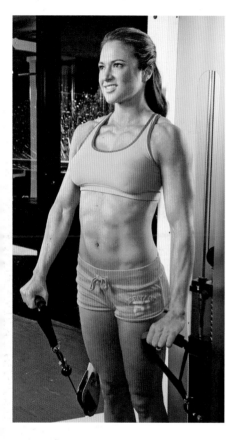

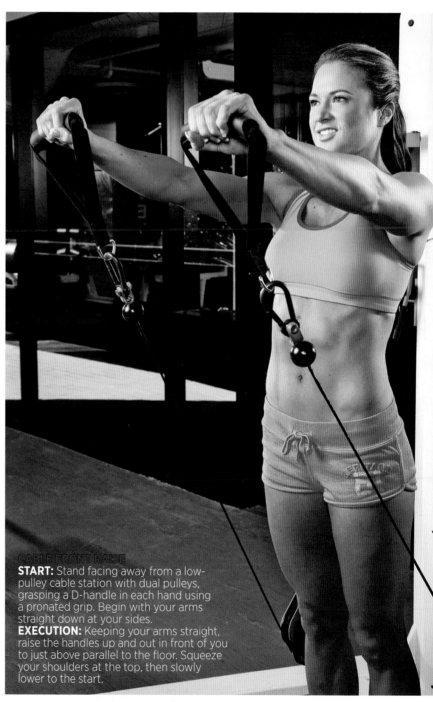

30-Minute Methods:
Supersets, high reps, variety

EXERCISE	SETS/REPS
Dumbbell Squat	2/20
—superset with—	
Overhead Dumbbell Press	2/20
Leg Extension	2/20
—superset with—	
Cable Front Raise	2/20
Leg Curl	2/20
—superset with—	
Lateral Raise	2/20
Cable Lunge	2/20
—superset with—	
Reverse Pec-deck Flye	2/20
Wall Squat with	
Static Lateral Raise	4/To failure

NOTE: During all supersets, rest only as long as it takes to set up for the next exercise. Rest as little as possible—no longer than 45 seconds—between all working sets.

CABLE FRONT RAISE

START: Stand facing away from a low-pulley cable station with dual pulleys, grasping a D-handle in each hand using a pronated grip. Begin with your arms straight down at your sides.
EXECUTION: Keeping your arms straight, raise the handles up and out in front of you to just above parallel to the floor. Squeeze your shoulders at the top, then slowly lower to the start.

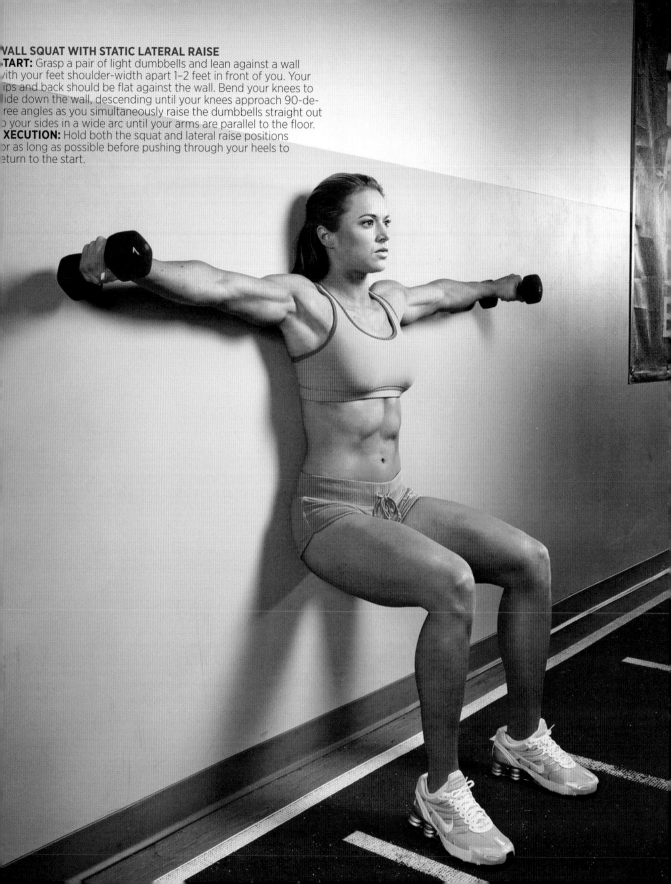

WALL SQUAT WITH STATIC LATERAL RAISE

START: Grasp a pair of light dumbbells and lean against a wall with your feet shoulder-width apart 1–2 feet in front of you. Your hips and back should be flat against the wall. Bend your knees to slide down the wall, descending until your knees approach 90-degree angles as you simultaneously raise the dumbbells straight out to your sides in a wide arc until your arms are parallel to the floor.

EXECUTION: Hold both the squat and lateral raise positions for as long as possible before pushing through your heels to return to the start.

Workout No.2:
BACK, HAMSTRINGS & GLUTES

You want to look just as good walking out of a room as you do walking in. That means paying due attention to your back, hamstrings, and glutes. Not surprisingly, these are among many people's least favorite body parts to train. The lifts require a lot of muscle and demand a great deal of energy. But hey, if you can crank through a killer routine for all these major muscle groups in just 30 minutes, then it becomes a lot more palatable, right?

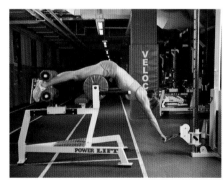

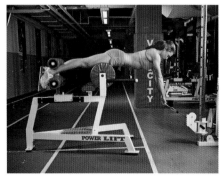

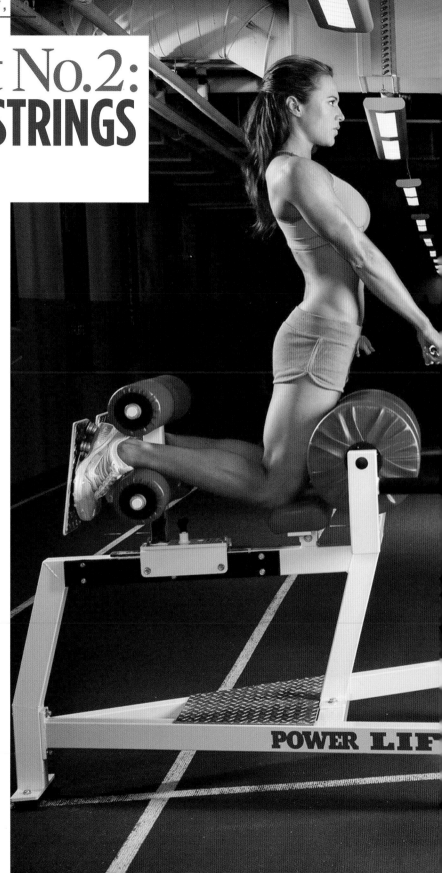

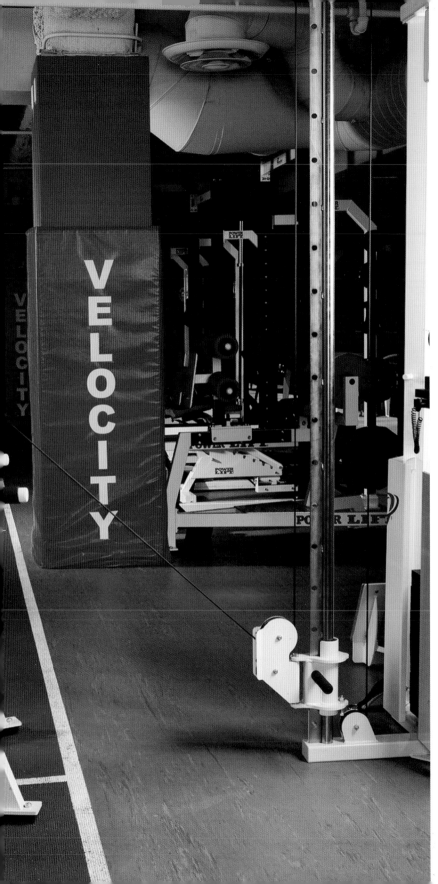

CABLE GLUTE-HAM RAISE

START: Set a back extension bench a few feet away from a cable station with the pulley at its lowest setting. Secure the backs of your ankles under the pad or rollers and place your thighs flush against the pad. Grasp the D-handle with both hands, arms extended, and begin with your torso just past parallel to the floor.

EXECUTION: Pull yourself up using your hamstrings and glutes until your body forms a straight line. From there, keep pulling yourself up slowly by bending your knees and raising your torso until it's perpendicular to the floor.

30-Minute Methods: Compound movements, low reps, high reps, variety

EXERCISE	SETS/REPS
Assisted Pullup	1/20–30*
Leg Curl	1/20–30*
Back Extension	1/20–30*
Romanian Deadlift	3/8–10
Cable Glute-ham Raise	2/10–12
Cable Straight-leg Kickback	2/12–15 per side
Seated Row	2/15–20
Assisted Pullup	1/To failure

Warmup set—do not take to failure.

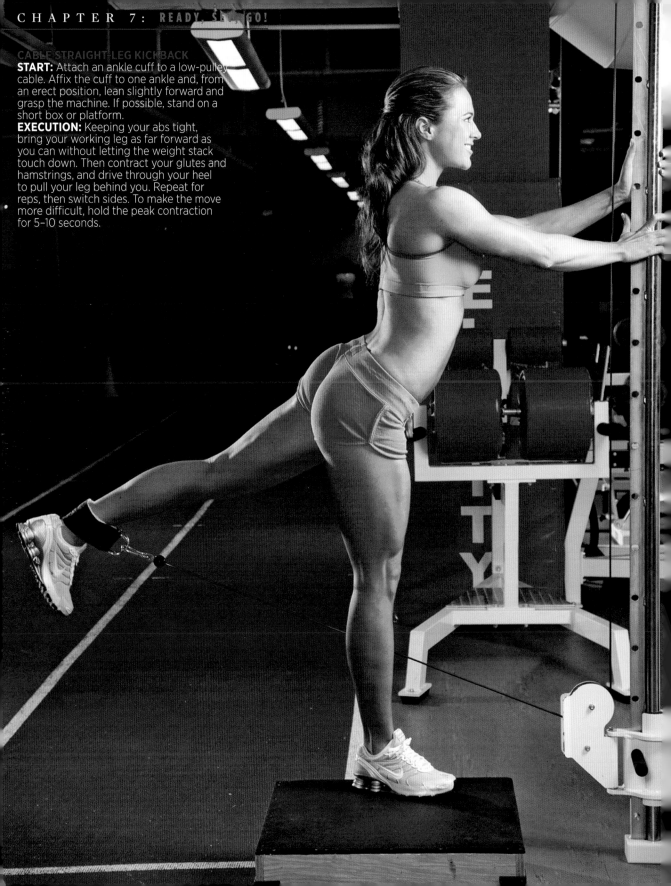

CABLE STRAIGHT-LEG KICKBACK

START: Attach an ankle cuff to a low-pulley cable. Affix the cuff to one ankle and, from an erect position, lean slightly forward and grasp the machine. If possible, stand on a short box or platform.

EXECUTION: Keeping your abs tight, bring your working leg as far forward as you can without letting the weight stack touch down. Then contract your glutes and hamstrings, and drive through your heel to pull your leg behind you. Repeat for reps, then switch sides. To make the move more difficult, hold the peak contraction for 5–10 seconds.

Workout No.3:
UPPER BODY & ABS

hough you want a stronger-looking upper body, you just don't have enough time (or ys in the week) to devote to chest, back, shoulders, biceps, triceps, and abs. Or do you? s routine, which employs similar movement patterns using supersets, puts all of those scle groups to the test in a very short amount of time. (Note: You could complete this rkout in about 15 minutes!) Every superset works through a similar plane in push/pull hion—for example, a lat pulldown followed by an overhead press. Training opposing scle groups back to back helps you stay strong throughout the routine, which is why s type of superset is a great idea for the time-crunched masses.

30-Minute Methods: Supersets, compound movements

EXERCISE	SETS/REPS
Lat Pulldown	2/12
—superset with—	
Overhead Press	2/12
Cable Front Raise	2/12
—superset with—	
Straight-Arm Lat Pulldown	2/12
Wide-Grip Seated Row	2/12
—superset with—	
Machine Chest Press	2/12
Cable Curl	2/12
—superset with—	
Incline Cable Triceps Extension	2/12
Double Crunch	2/To failure

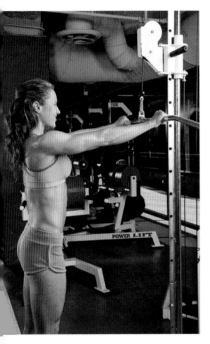

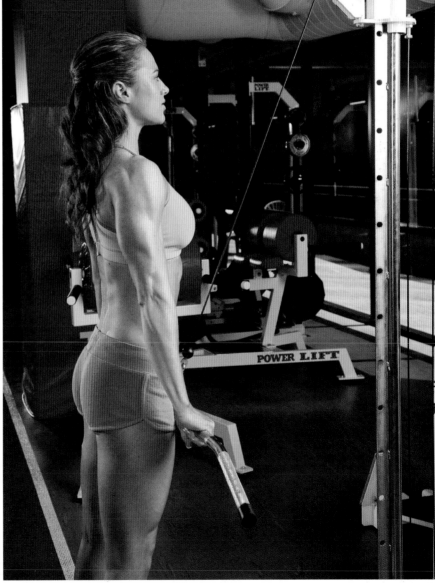

RAIGHT-ARM LAT PULLDOWN
ART: Stand facing the weight stack ng a shoulder-width stance. Grasp the aight bar with an overhand grip, hands ulder width. Begin with the bar at ulder level, arms extended.
ECUTION: Pull the bar toward your ghs in a wide arc, focusing on using just ur lats. Squeeze your lats hard, then urn in a smooth, controlled motion, pping when your arms come parallel the floor.

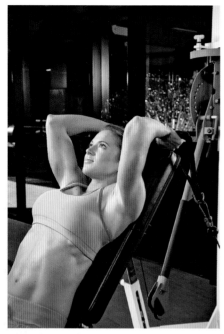

INCLINE CABLE TRICEPS EXTENSION

START: Position an incline bench facing away from a cable stack. Attach a bar or two handles to the lowest pulley setting. Grasp the bar or handles and sit back on the bench with your arms extended straight up toward the ceiling.

EXECUTION: Bend your elbows to lower your hands down and behind your head, keeping your upper arms stationary throughout. When your elbows reach 90 degrees, contract your triceps to extend your arms back to the start position.

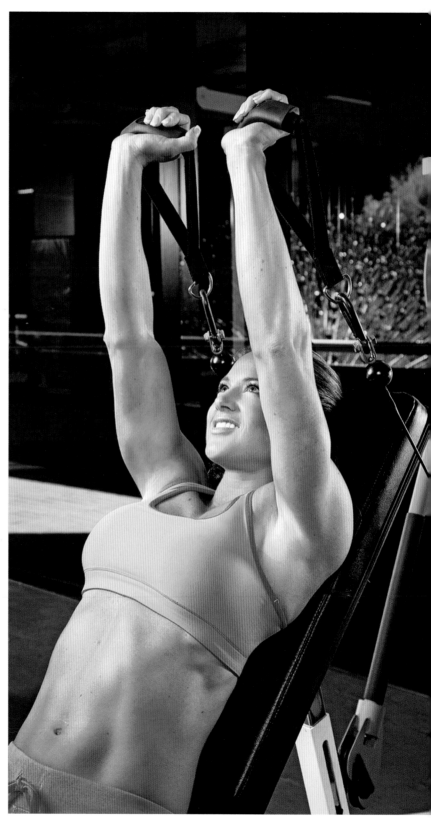

Workout No.4:
WHOLE BODY

Looking to get a quick full-body burn before drowning in a deluge of holiday ham, sweet potatoes, stuffing, and cheesecake? We've got just the thing. This 30-minute blast hits your entire body with a variety of movements, angles, and equipment. The payoff is a head-to-toe workout that builds strength, burns fat, and increases athleticism.

30-Minute Methods: Compound movements, variety

EXERCISE	SETS/REPS
Dumbbell Deadlift to Step-Up* to Overhead Press	4/10
Lunge with Medicine Ball Twist	3/16 steps
Medicine Ball Swing	3/15 per side
Squat Jump	3/15
Speed Skater	3/To failure
Pushup**	2/To failure

*Alternate legs each rep.
**Complete as many standard pushups as you can. When you can no longer perform those, drop to your knees and rep to failure.

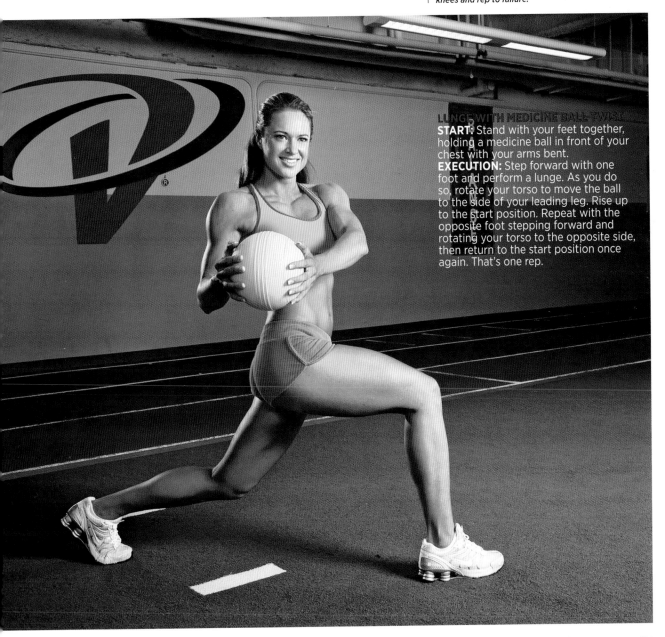

LUNGE WITH MEDICINE BALL TWIST
START: Stand with your feet together, holding a medicine ball in front of your chest with your arms bent.
EXECUTION: Step forward with one foot and perform a lunge. As you do so, rotate your torso to move the ball to the side of your leading leg. Rise up to the start position. Repeat with the opposite foot stepping forward and rotating your torso to the opposite side, then return to the start position once again. That's one rep.

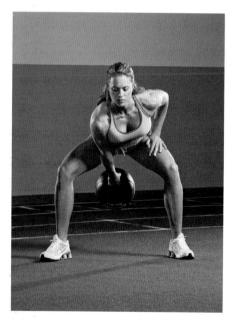

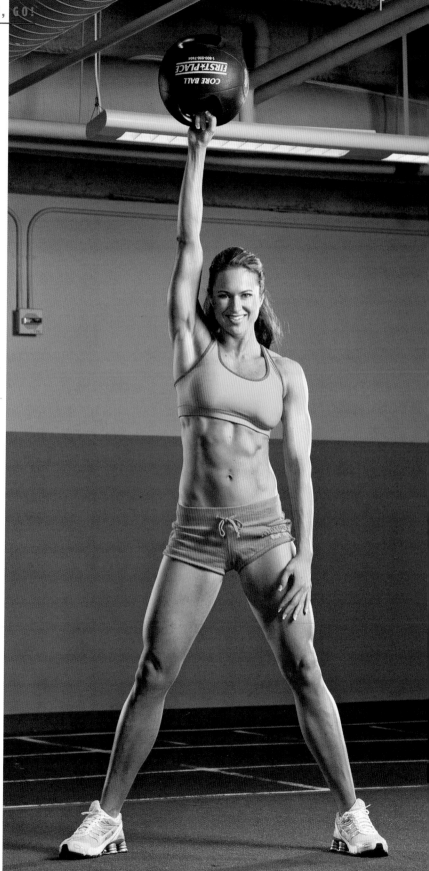

MEDICINE-BALL SWING

START: Stand with your feet wider than shoulder-width apart with a weighted ball on the floor between them. Squat down to grasp the ball using a palms-down grip. Lean forward 45 degrees with your arm tensed and pulling on the ball, your thighs slightly above parallel to the floor.

EXECUTION: In one smooth motion, forcefully extend your hips and knees as you swing the ball forward and up in a wide arc until it's directly overhead. Immediately squat back down to the start position, allowing the weight to swing down and back along the same arc until it's once again beneath you. Repeat for reps, then switch sides.

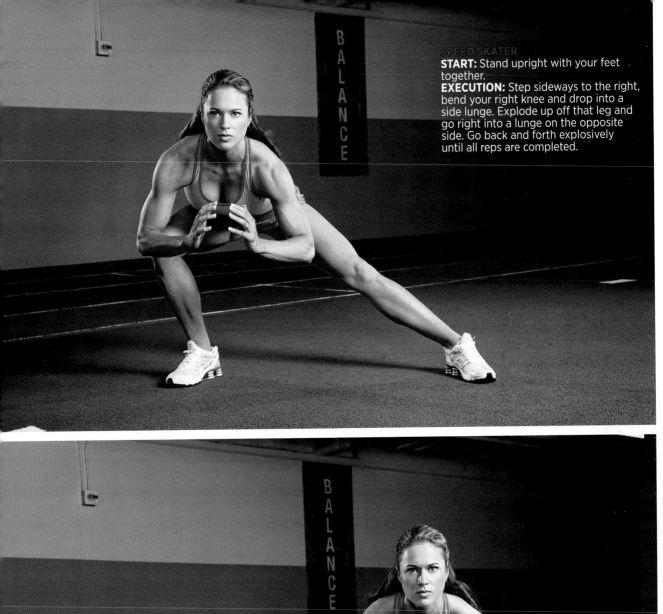

SPEED SKATER

START: Stand upright with your feet together.
EXECUTION: Step sideways to the right, bend your right knee and drop into a side lunge. Explode up off that leg and go right into a lunge on the opposite side. Go back and forth explosively until all reps are completed.

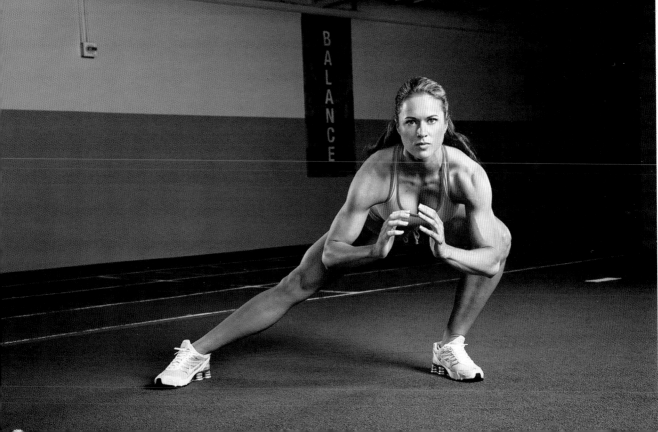

CHAPTER 8

RAISE THE BAR

Achieve a sleek, toned body with these Olympic lifting classics

They're fun, easy to learn, highly efficient, and not just for elite athletes anymore. Olympic lifts such as the snatch and clean offer the best bang for your buck in the gym, and if you're serious about going after the body you want, you need to learn them. With just a few moves you can work every muscle group, burn fat, and train your cardiovascular system—all in very little time.

Olympic lifters have lean, strong muscles; and training for power burns more calories and produces better muscular development for women who want an athletic physique. In addition, research from the U.S. Olympic Training Center found that subjects who incorporated Olympic lifts into their routines performed better on the vertical jump and improved their cardiovascular fitness.

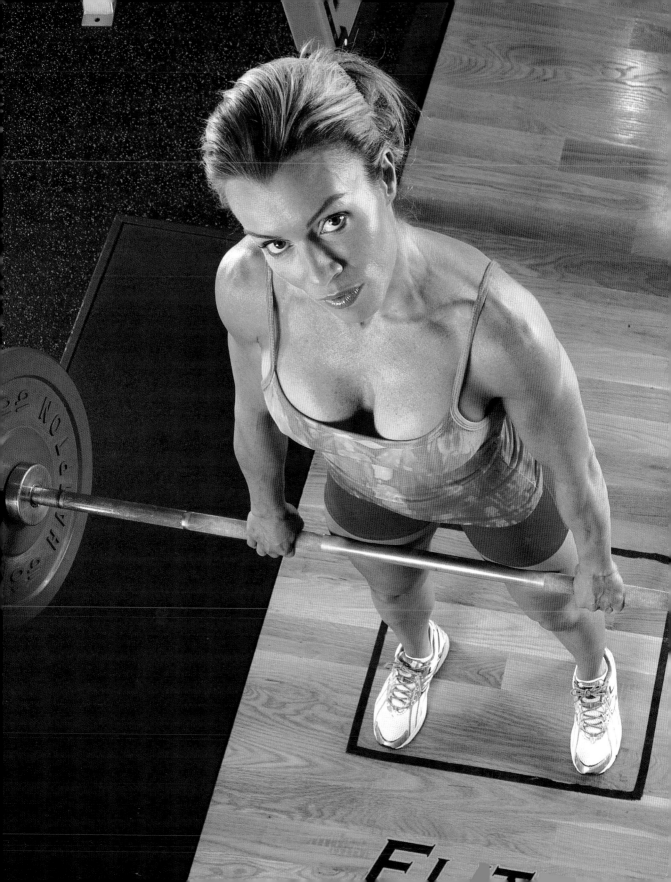

This program will serve as an introduction to Olympic-style training. After 12 weeks you'll be able to push a loaded bar overhead and land in a position that works your core like nothing you've ever experienced in the gym.

To do this workout properly, you'll need access to specific equipment. Because you'll use all your power performing the moves, it'll be difficult to slowly and safely set the bar back on the floor. We suggest using rubber tiles on a specially designed platform so you can drop the weight to the floor after you complete a rep. If your gym doesn't have these, perform the move carefully and catch the bar on your shoulders before lowering it.

Since you might not be familiar with these exercises, you'll likely start off with too little weight. This can be problematic because using reasonably heavy weight helps you perform the moves correctly. The barbell has to be heavy enough that you use your entire body to lift it. If it's too light, you might try to move it using just a couple of muscle groups, and attempting to get a loaded bar overhead using only your deltoids, for example, is a shortcut to injury. As soon as you become comfortable with these lifts, add weight to the bar.

These moves require a lot of power. If you do them correctly—giving all you've got—you won't be able to perform high-rep sets. Your power will diminish with each rep and your form will begin to deteriorate. This can also lead to injury, so keep your rep ranges low and intense, generating as much power as you can for no more than 6–8 reps. Recover fully between sets.

The Program

In Phase 1 you'll start with higher rep ranges as you practice the fundamental movements: pressing the bar overhead as you squat, exploding a load up using momentum rather than just your arms, and getting comfortable doing a front squat.

Next, you'll learn the first cornerstone Olympic movement: the clean. You'll also begin pressing a barbell overhead explosively, and continue to strengthen your front squat using lower reps and more weight. Phase 3 will address two more principal moves: the snatch and the clean to split jerk. Note that this program doesn't call for more than eight reps in any set. In fact, the number of reps you'll perform will decrease as you incorporate the Olympic lifts. With each set you'll add weight and develop confidence.

THE WORKOUT

PHASE 1

EXERCISE	SETS	REPS	REST
Pressing Snatch Balance	2–4	6–8	45–60 sec.
High Pull	2–4	6–8	45–60 sec.
Front Squat	2–4	6–8	45–60 sec.

PHASE 2

EXERCISE	SETS	REPS	REST
Clean	2–4	4–6	60–90 sec.
Push Press	2–4	4–6	60–90 sec.
Front Squat	2–4	4–6	60–90 sec.

PHASE 3

EXERCISE	SETS	REPS	REST
High Pull	2–4	2–4	90–120 sec.
Snatch	2–4	5,4,3,2	90–120 sec.
Clean to Split Jerk	2–4	5,4,3,2	90–120 sec.

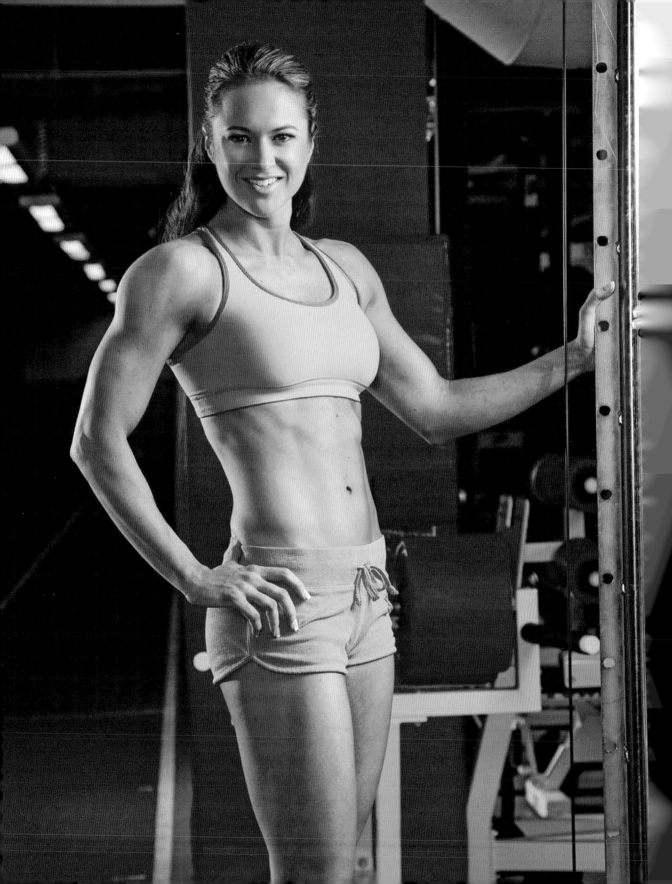

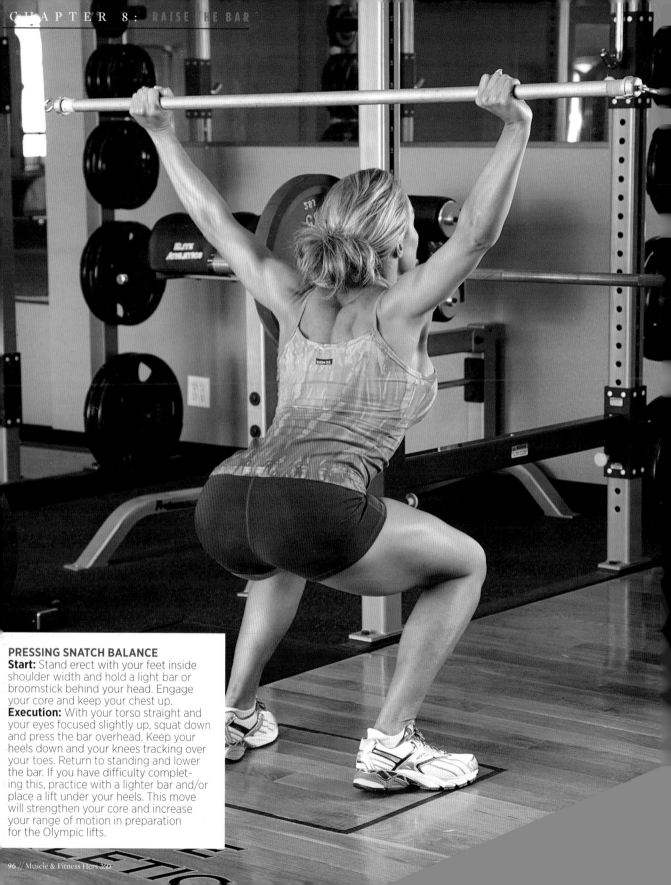

PRESSING SNATCH BALANCE

Start: Stand erect with your feet inside shoulder width and hold a light bar or broomstick behind your head. Engage your core and keep your chest up.

Execution: With your torso straight and your eyes focused slightly up, squat down and press the bar overhead. Keep your heels down and your knees tracking over your toes. Return to standing and lower the bar. If you have difficulty completing this, practice with a lighter bar and/or place a lift under your heels. This move will strengthen your core and increase your range of motion in preparation for the Olympic lifts.

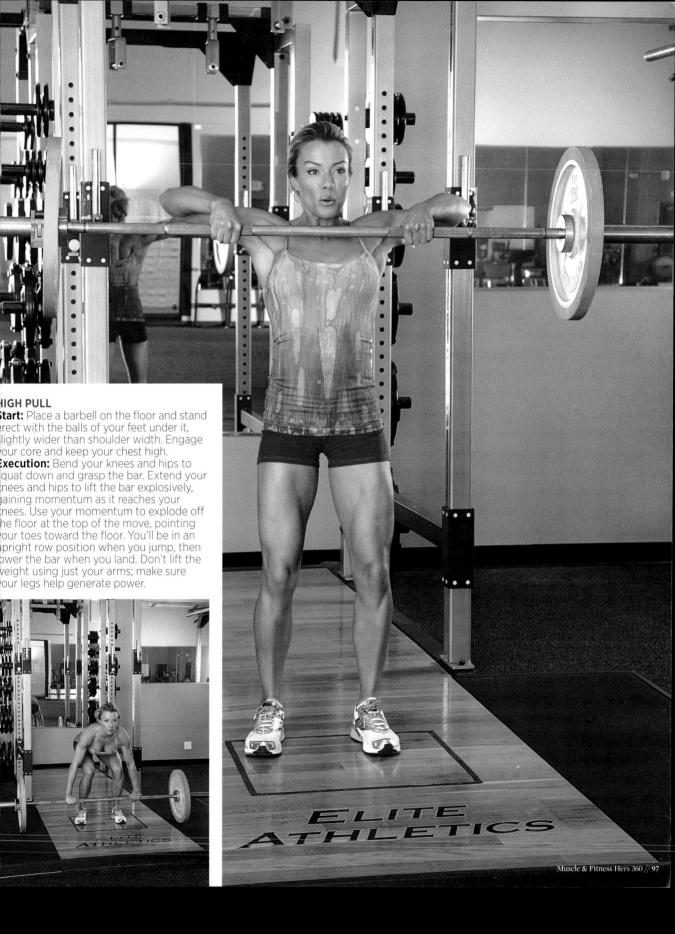

HIGH PULL

Start: Place a barbell on the floor and stand erect with the balls of your feet under it, slightly wider than shoulder width. Engage your core and keep your chest high.

Execution: Bend your knees and hips to squat down and grasp the bar. Extend your knees and hips to lift the bar explosively, gaining momentum as it reaches your knees. Use your momentum to explode off the floor at the top of the move, pointing your toes toward the floor. You'll be in an upright row position when you jump, then lower the bar when you land. Don't lift the weight using just your arms; make sure your legs help generate power.

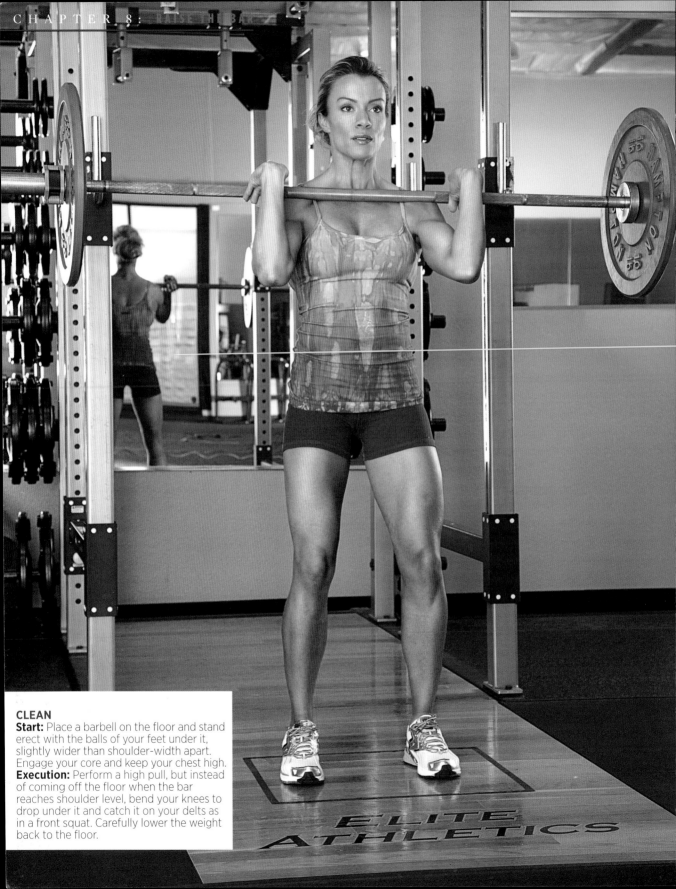

CLEAN

Start: Place a barbell on the floor and stand erect with the balls of your feet under it, slightly wider than shoulder-width apart. Engage your core and keep your chest high.

Execution: Perform a high pull, but instead of coming off the floor when the bar reaches shoulder level, bend your knees to drop under it and catch it on your delts as in a front squat. Carefully lower the weight back to the floor.

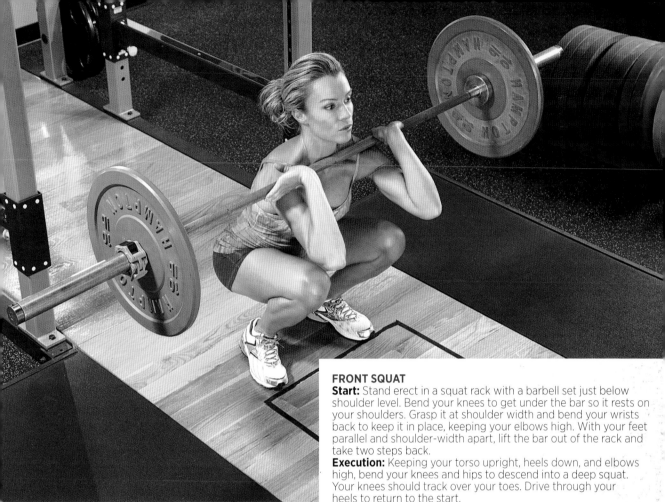

FRONT SQUAT

Start: Stand erect in a squat rack with a barbell set just below shoulder level. Bend your knees to get under the bar so it rests on your shoulders. Grasp it at shoulder width and bend your wrists back to keep it in place, keeping your elbows high. With your feet parallel and shoulder-width apart, lift the bar out of the rack and take two steps back.

Execution: Keeping your torso upright, heels down, and elbows high, bend your knees and hips to descend into a deep squat. Your knees should track over your toes. Drive through your heels to return to the start.

PUSH PRESS

Start: Stand erect in a squat rack with a barbell set just below shoulder level. Bend your knees to get under the bar so it rests on your shoulders. Grasp it at shoulder width and bend your wrists back to keep it in place, keeping your elbows high, as in the front squat. With your feet parallel and shoulder-width apart, lift the bar out of the rack and take two steps back.

Execution: Bend your knees and hips slightly, then push off the floor and simultaneously press the bar overhead, using power from your legs and hips. Catch the weight by locking your shoulders and elbows. Engage your core for support and keep your knees slightly bent. Don't try to muscle the bar down; instead, let it land on your shoulders, bending your knees as you catch it.

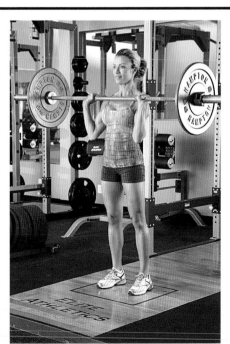
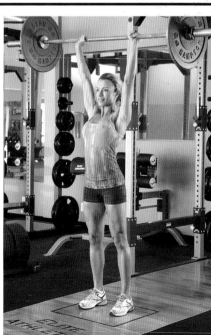

SNATCH

Start: Place a barbell on the floor and stand erect with the balls of your feet under it, slightly wider than shoulder-width apart. Engage your core and keep your chest high.

Execution: Bend your knees and hips to squat down and grasp the bar. Extend your knees and hips to lift the bar explosively, gaining momentum as it reaches your knees. Instead of stopping the weight at chest level as you did in the high pull and clean, continue accelerating to explode the bar overhead. Drop under the weight, keeping it above and slightly behind your head, then extend your knees to return to standing before slowly lowering the bar.

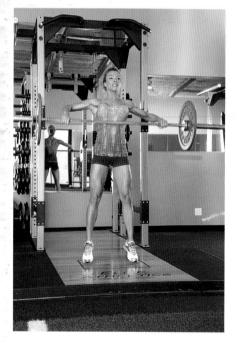

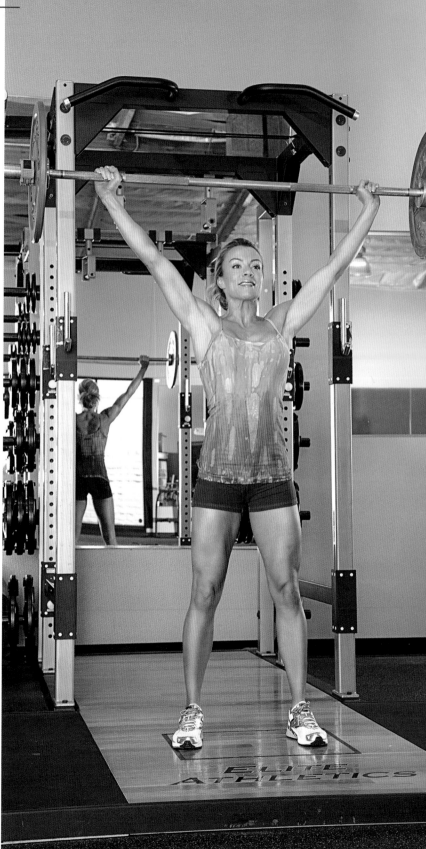

LEAN TO SPLIT JERK

Start: Place a barbell on the floor and stand erect with the balls of your feet under it, slightly wider than shoulder-width apart. Engage your core and keep your chest high.

Execution: Perform a clean. With the bar in front squat position, explode the weight overhead and land in a split stance with your knees bent, your core engaged and your chest high. If you're uncomfortable with this move, practice with an empty bar. To return to the start, bring your back foot forward, then lower the weight.

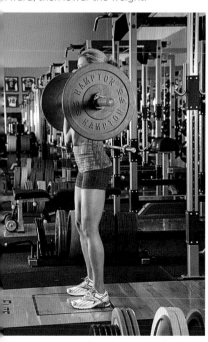

CHAPTER 9

LOSE POUNDS WITH PLYO

This workout can be performed one of two ways—with fewer sets, more reps, and less rest for conditioning; or with more sets, fewer reps, and more rest for a strength workout. Keep an eye out for these bursts, which will tell you what to do based on the type of exercise you're looking for.

Fire up your metabolism and shed pounds with an intense plyometrics workout. This all-in-one training technique, demonstrated by IFBB bikini pro Tawna Eubanks, uses explosive movements to power up your fat-burning cylinders (and enhance bone density). Here, we give you five moves that build strength, agility, and a sexy midsection and lower body—fast.

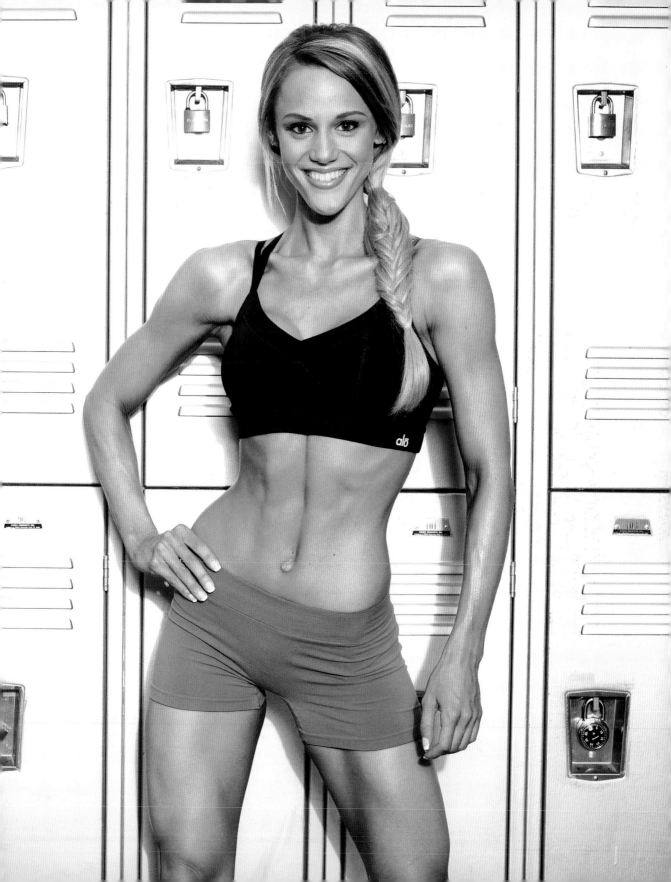

Bulgarian Lunge

SETS, REPS, REST
CONDITIONING: 3–5x15
no rest, alternating legs
STRENGTH: 6x6
rest 2 min.

Works: Shoulders, Core, Glutes, Hamstrings, Quads

• Holding a dumbbell in each hand, stand lunge-distance from a box or flat bench, facing away from it.
• Place the top of your foot on the box.
• Keeping your chest up and your front foot flat, slowly lower straight down into a lunge position until your front thigh is at least parallel to the floor.
• Drive through your front heel to return to standing.

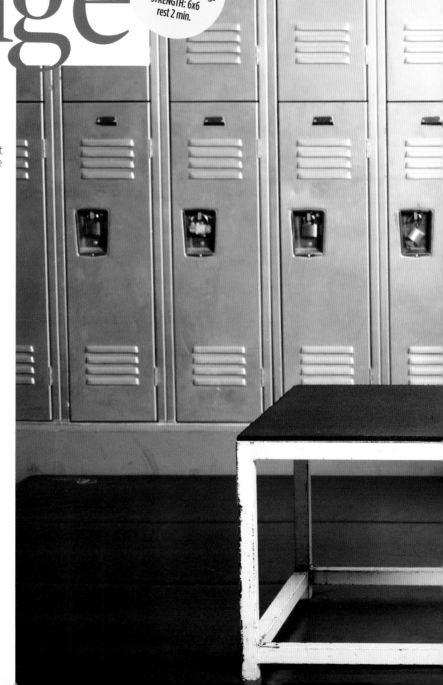

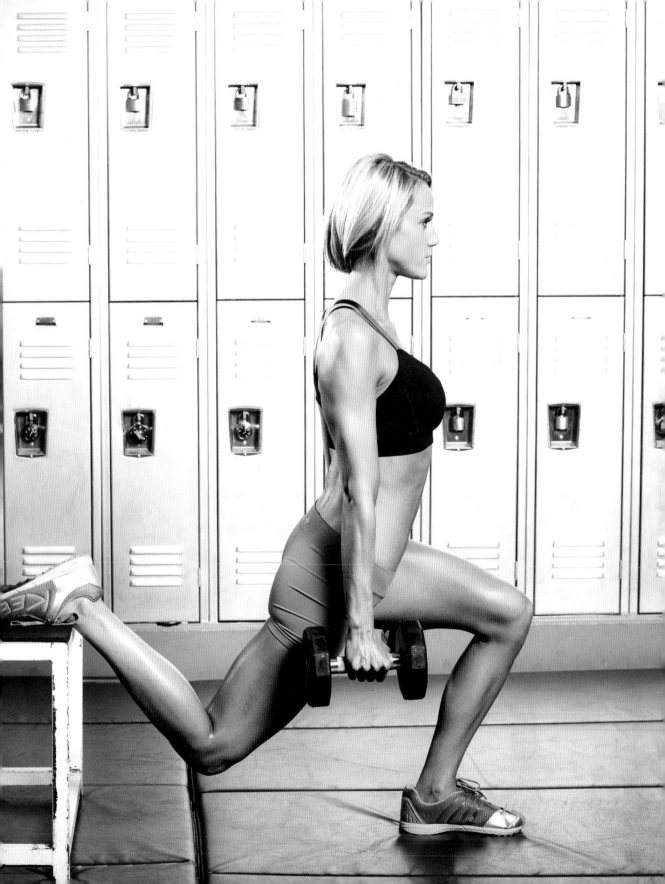

Single-Leg Step-Up with Knee Drive

Works: Glutes, Hamstrings, Quads

• Holding a dumbbell in each hand, stand with your left side next to a flat bench and place your left foot (your driving leg) on top of it.
• Push through the center of your driving foot, pressing your body straight up onto the bench while lifting your right leg to a 90-degree angle.
• Reverse the motion to step back down, repeat.

SETS, REPS, REST
CONDITIONING: 4x12 rest 90 sec.
STRENGTH: 6x6 rest 2 min.

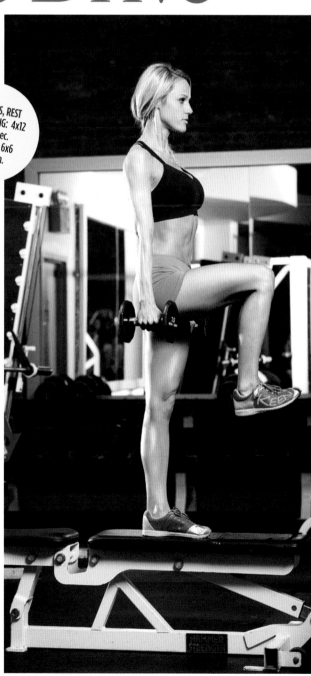

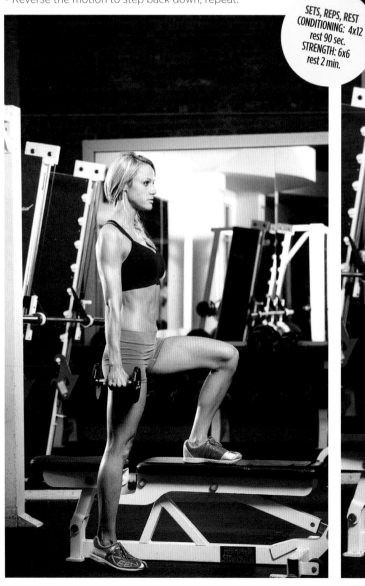

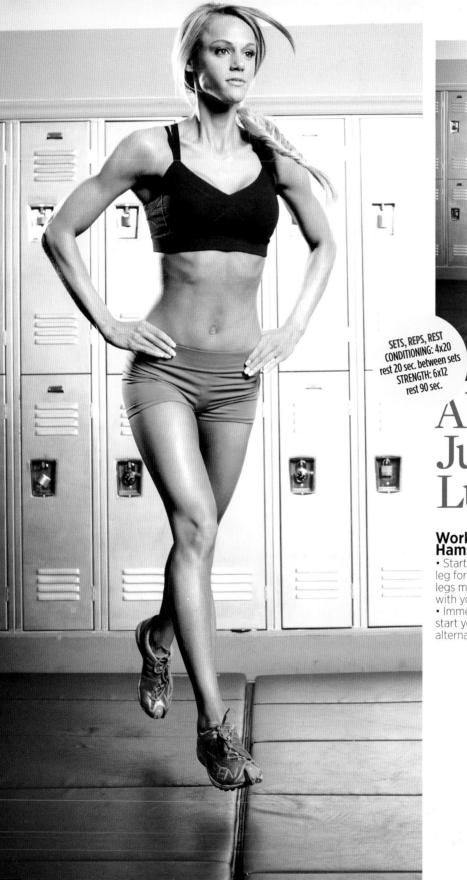

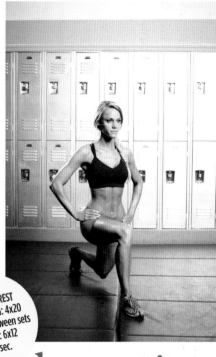

SETS, REPS, REST
CONDITIONING: 4x20
rest 20 sec. between sets
STRENGTH: 6x12
rest 90 sec.

Alternating Jump Lunge

Works: Core, Glutes, Hamstrings, Quads, Calves

• Starting in a lunge position with your left leg forward, jump straight up and switch legs midair, landing softly in lunge position with your right leg forward.

• Immediately push off after landing to start your next jump, continuing to alternate legs.

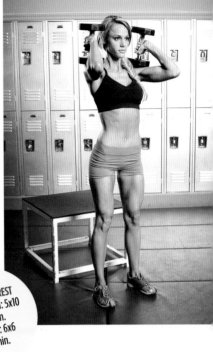

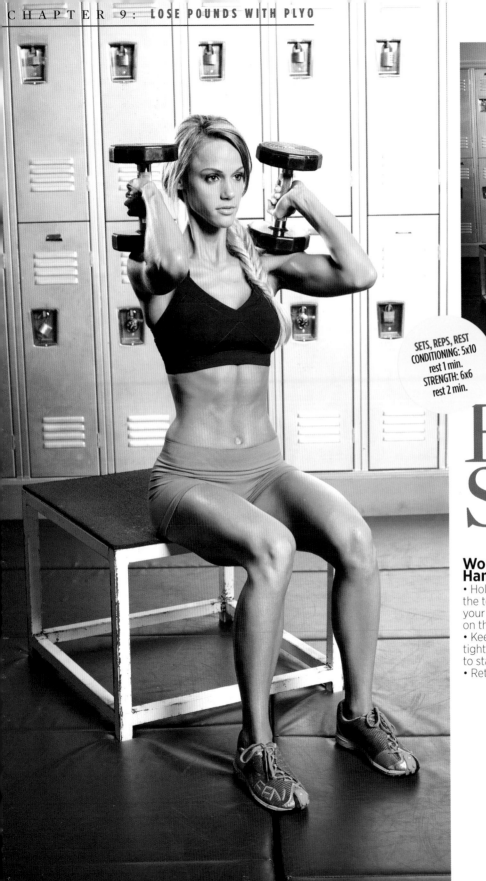

SETS, REPS, REST
CONDITIONING: 5x10
rest 1 min.
STRENGTH: 6x6
rest 2 min.

Box Squat

Works: Core, Glutes, Hamstrings, Quads

• Holding a dumbbell in each hand, with the tops resting on your shoulders and your upper arms parallel to the floor, sit on the edge of a box or flat bench.
• Keeping your chest up and midsection tight, drive through your heels to come to standing.
• Return to sitting and then repeat.

Single-Leg Squat

orks: Glutes, Hamstrings

tand in a Smith machine, grip the barbell with your right hand,
d hold a dumbbell in your left hand.
aise your left leg off the floor, foot flexed, and sink down into a
uat until your right thigh is at least parallel to the floor.
rive through your heel to push up to the starting position.

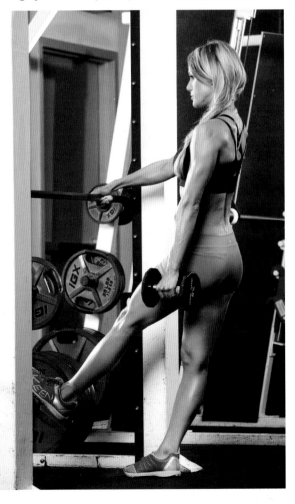

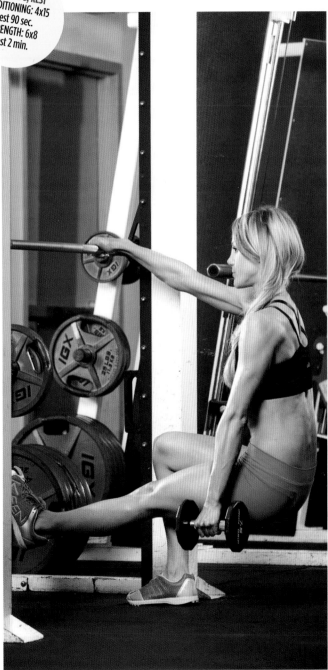

CHAPTER 10

YOGA
FOR FIT CHICKS

Want a body that looks this good? Maybe it's time to finally give yoga a try. As demonstrated here by IFBB fitness pro Bethany Cisternino, these postures not only work every muscle while stretching you out—they'll also help keep your mind clear while getting your body fit and strong.

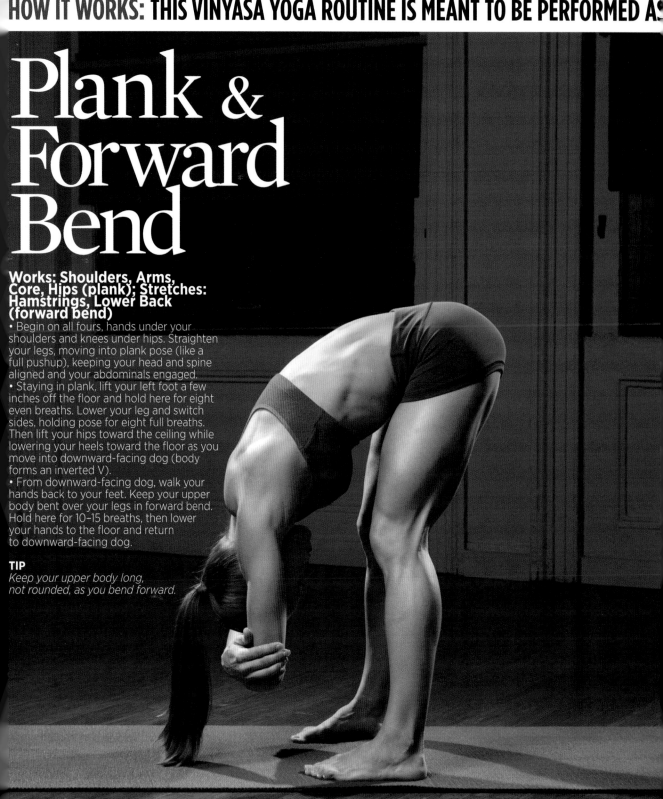

HOW IT WORKS: THIS VINYASA YOGA ROUTINE IS MEANT TO BE PERFORMED AS

Plank & Forward Bend

Works: Shoulders, Arms, Core, Hips (plank); Stretches: Hamstrings, Lower Back (forward bend)

• Begin on all fours, hands under your shoulders and knees under hips. Straighten your legs, moving into plank pose (like a full pushup), keeping your head and spine aligned and your abdominals engaged.

• Staying in plank, lift your left foot a few inches off the floor and hold here for eight even breaths. Lower your leg and switch sides, holding pose for eight full breaths. Then lift your hips toward the ceiling while lowering your heels toward the floor as you move into downward-facing dog (body forms an inverted V).

• From downward-facing dog, walk your hands back to your feet. Keep your upper body bent over your legs in forward bend. Hold here for 10–15 breaths, then lower your hands to the floor and return to downward-facing dog.

TIP
Keep your upper body long, not rounded, as you bend forward.

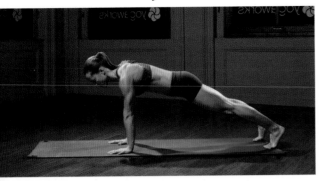

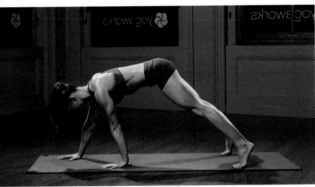

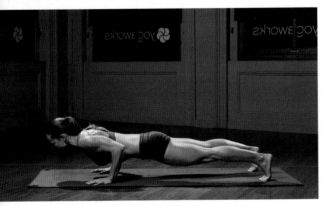

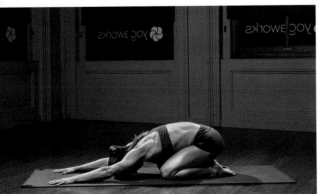

Yoga Pushup & Child's Pose

Works: Shoulders, Triceps, Core, Thighs (pushup); Stretches: Shoulders, Arms, Back, Hips (child's pose)

• From downward dog, shift forward to plank pose. Bend your elbows, keeping your arms close to your sides as you lower half-way down into yoga pushup (chaturanga).

• Straighten your arms, pressing your hands into the floor to move back to plank pose (not shown). Repeat yoga pushup/plank sequence 10 times.

• After final pushup, press hips back toward ceiling to downward-facing dog. Stay here for one breath, then bring knees to the floor, sitting back on your feet and reaching for-ward with your arms as you rest in child's pose. Repeat one more set of yoga pushup/plank series.

TIP
Keep elbows hugged close to sides of your body and abs pulled in during the yoga pushup.

Crow

Works: Arms, Abs, Hips

• Bring palms flat onto floor, about shoulder-width apart, and squat down, keeping your feet and hands close.
• Lifting your feet off the floor one at a time, place your knees onto the back of your upper arms. Draw your navel toward your spine and hold.

TIP
To make crow easier, bend your elbows and push firmly into hands.

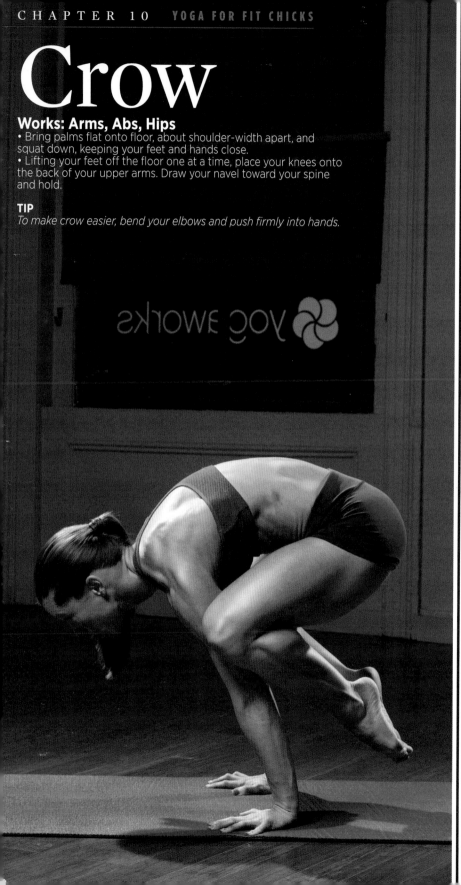

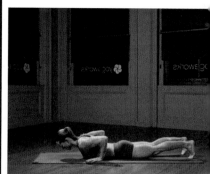

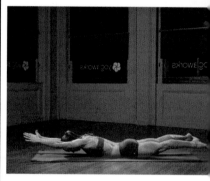

Grasshoppe

Works: Shoulders, Lower Bacl Thighs

• Begin in plank. Do one yoga pushup, keeping elbows close to your sides. Lowe your body all the way to floor.
• Reach both arms forward, palms facing each other, while lifting your chest and legs. Stay here for 15 breaths.
• Lower chest and legs to floor then repea series from plank two more times. To finis bring hands back to mat and press halfwa up to yoga push-up. Continue pressing ur into plank pose, arms straight, then raise hips toward ceiling as you move into downward facing dog.

TIP
While in grasshopper, extend arms forwar while reaching back with heels.

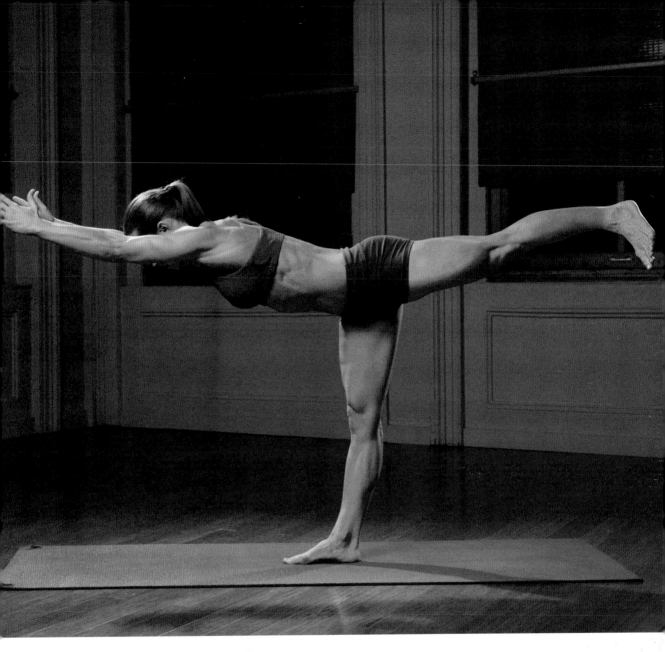

Warrior 3

Works: Shoulders, Arms, Core, Back, Glutes, Thighs; Balance

• From downward-facing dog, lift left leg to hip height. Walk hands back, keeping left leg lifted, then rise up, extending arms next to your ears with palms facing each other. Hold for 10–15 breaths, reaching forward with your arms and back with your left leg.

• Lower hands to the floor and walk them back out to downward dog, lowering your right leg to the floor. Repeat sequence on left side, ending in downward facing dog.

TIP

Keep hips level and square to the floor while pulling your belly in for support.

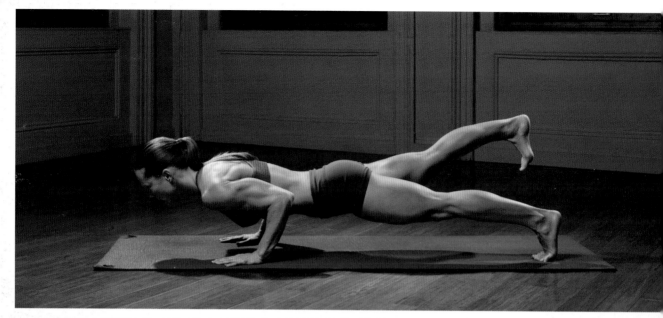

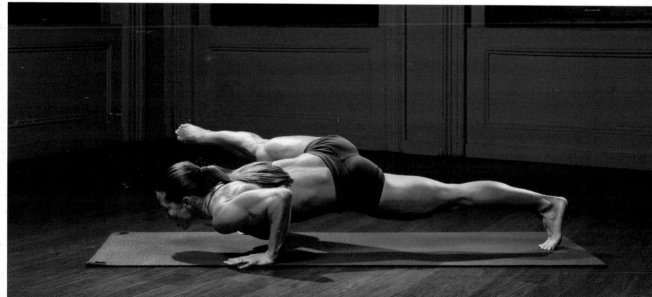

Yoga Pushup Series

Works: Shoulders, Triceps, Core, Glutes, Thighs, Calves

• From downward dog, shift your weight forward to move into plank pose. Lower halfway to yoga pushup. Lift your right foot and hold here for five breaths.

• Lower your right foot to the floor briefly, then bring your right foot as far as you can out to the right, keeping your leg straight; hold here for five breaths.

• Return foot to center, keeping it lifted, and press to downward dog. Lower your right leg to floor. Shift to plank and repeat low pushup series with left leg, ending in downward dog.

TIP

Keep shoulders level and square to mat, don't allow your lower back to sag.

Boat & Half Boat

Works: Shoulders, Biceps, Abs, Thighs

Sit on the floor, legs extended forward and arms at your sides. Reach arms forward at shoulder height while lifting both legs 45 degrees to floor, forming a V. Lower into half boat, bringing your legs and upper body toward the floor; keep your head, neck, shoulders, and legs lifted while continuing to reach forward. Come up to full boat, then lower again to half boat. Repeat sequence 10 times; rest a few moments and repeat for another 10 reps.

TIP

Keep chest open and legs together, spreading toes as you reach legs forward.

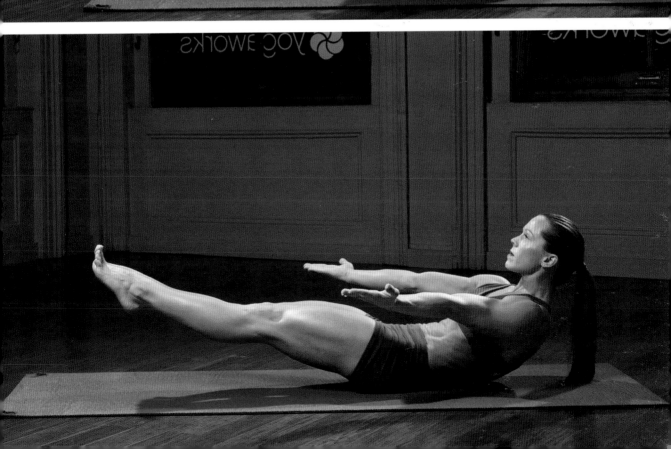

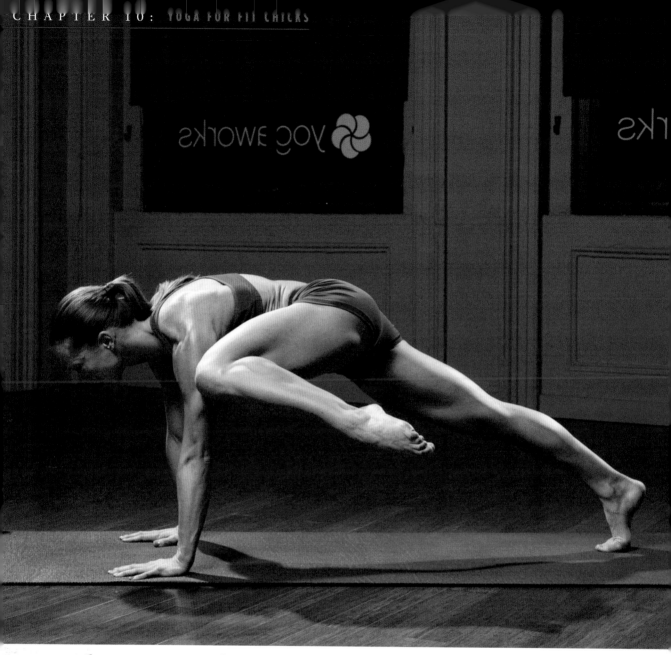

Plank Pull-in

Works: Shoulders, Arms, Core, Back, Glutes, Thighs, Calves

• From downward-facing dog, shift forward to plank pose. Pull left knee to back of left triceps, rounding your back while keeping arms straight. Hold pose for five breaths.

• Lower your knee halfway to your elbow as you exhale. Inhale, pulling your leg back toward the top of your left arm.

• Repeat sequence five times, then return to downward-facing dog. Repeat full sequence with right leg.

TIP
Draw navel in and keep your elbows straight but not locked.

Handstand

Works: Shoulders, Core; Balance

• Begin in downward dog, then walk your feet forward, keeping your arms straight. Lift your right leg and hop up off left foot a few times to get your momentum going, then lift both feet off the floor as you move into a full handstand. Stay here as long as is comfortable.

TIP

To make it easier, practice handstands near a wall, keeping feet against wall for balance.

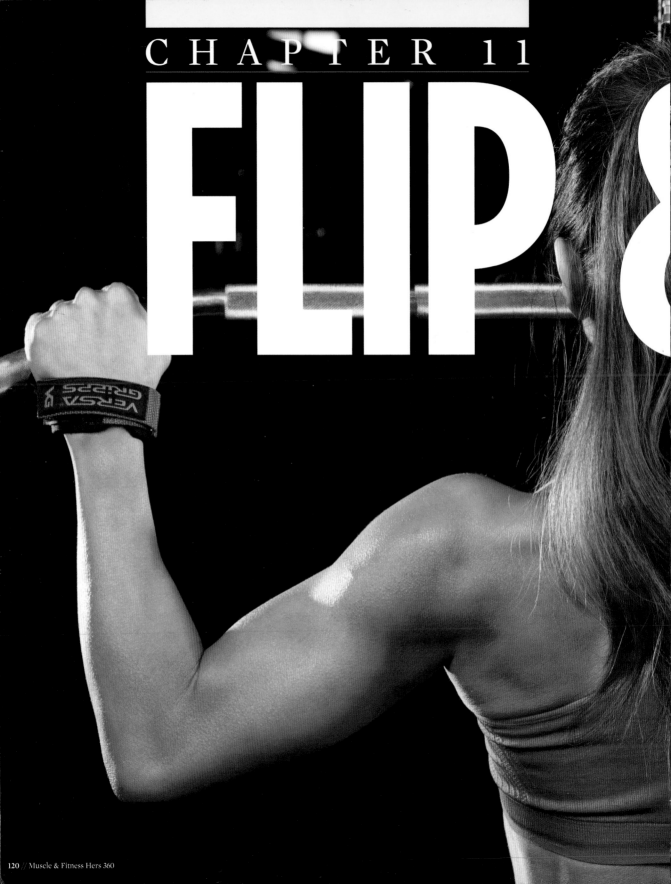

CHAPTER 11

FLIP &

GRIP

Training (and gains) a little ho-hum? Add these seven moves to your routine and flip back to growth.

For better or worse, we're creatures of habit. When we get used to something, we stick with it. You know, like that workout you do day in and day out, performing the same exercises in the exact same way. Well, some routines are meant to be broken. To keep that rut of yours from setting down roots and strangling your progress, you'll need to put some spring back in your training. That's where we come in. Here, we show you how to change your grip on commonly used exercises, from top to bottom. Yep, even the slightest change, such as handgrip position, can turn your muscle gains around. Now go on, flip off!

BACK

SAMPLE BACK WORKOUT

EXERCISE	SETS	REPS
Reverse-grip Lat Pulldown*	5	10–12
Reverse-grip Barbell Row	3–4	8–10
Close-grip Pulldown	3–4	8–10
Close-grip Cable Row	3	10–12

Includes two warmup sets of 12–15 reps each.

CLOSE-GRIP PULLDOWN

FOCUS AREA: LOWER LATS

ON THE FLIP SIDE: Granted, the pulldown is generally touted for being a hefty back-widening exercise. But if you're looking to add thickness to your back, close-grip (with hands close) movements are the way to go. With this grip, your elbows stay closer to your body, allowing you to generate more power, so you can lift heavier and better stimulate the lower lat muscle.

DIRECTIONS:
-Attach a close-grip cable attachment on lat pulldown machine. Grasp the handles.
-With your arms fully extended overhead, keep your abs tight, back slightly arched, and feet flat on the floor.
-Squeeze your shoulder blades together and pull the attachment toward your upper chest, keeping your elbows down and back.
-Squeeze and hold for a brief count before slowly allowing the attachment to return to start. Repeat for reps.

TIP:
Hold your elbows tight along your body as you pull the bar down toward your chest.

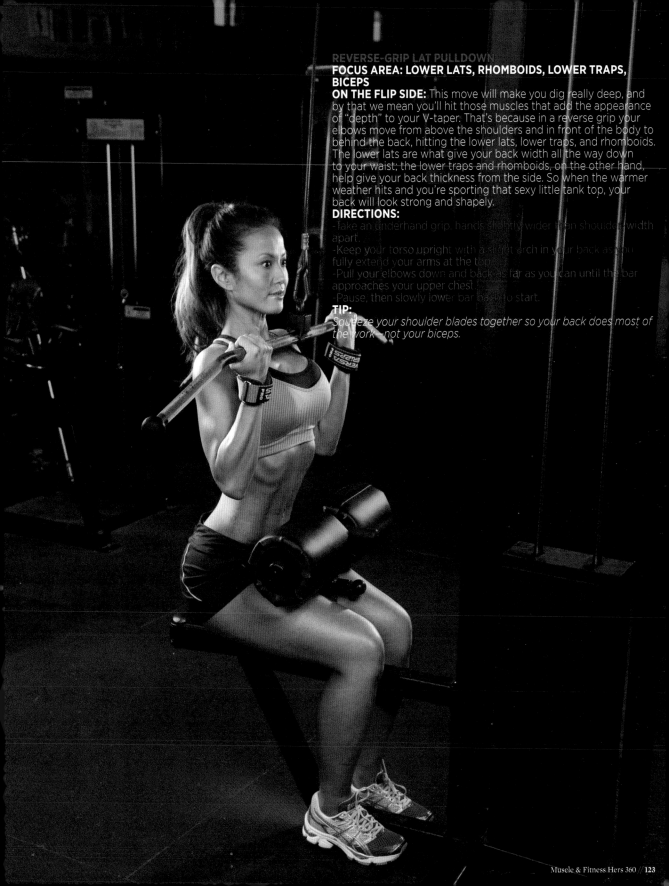

REVERSE-GRIP LAT PULLDOWN
FOCUS AREA: LOWER LATS, RHOMBOIDS, LOWER TRAPS, BICEPS

ON THE FLIP SIDE: This move will make you dig really deep, and by that we mean you'll hit those muscles that add the appearance of "depth" to your V-taper. That's because in a reverse grip your elbows move from above the shoulders and in front of the body to behind the back, hitting the lower lats, lower traps, and rhomboids. The lower lats are what give your back width all the way down to your waist; the lower traps and rhomboids, on the other hand, help give your back thickness from the side. So when the warmer weather hits and you're sporting that sexy little tank top, your back will look strong and shapely.

DIRECTIONS:
- Take an underhand grip, hands slightly wider than shoulder-width apart.
- Keep your torso upright with a slight arch in your back as you fully extend your arms at the top.
- Pull your elbows down and back as far as you can until the bar approaches your upper chest.
- Pause, then slowly lower bar back to start.

TIP:
Squeeze your shoulder blades together so your back does most of the work—not your biceps.

SAMPLE CHEST WORKOUT

EXERCISE	SETS	REPS
Barbell Bench Press*	5	8-10
Reverse-grip Incline Press	3	10-12
Neutral-grip Dumbbell Incline Press	3	12
Pec Deck	3	8-12

*Includes two warmup sets of 15 reps each.

CHEST

NEUTRAL-GRIP DUMBBELL INCLINE PRESS
FOCUS AREA: CHEST

ON THE FLIP SIDE: We understand if a monster bench press isn't at the top of your list of goals for the month. But you don't have to be breaking records to want better stimulation. Fact is, when the bar is at your chest, you've hit a sticky spot. This is where a neutral grip can help you push through your trouble zone. To gain strength, you need to train at your weakest point. And in this case, your weakest point is your chest. That's because barbell-pressing movements also involve the delts and triceps. When your palms are facing each other, however, your elbows tend to remain closer to your sides, so you remove the delts and triceps from the equation and place the emphasis where it's needed—your chest.

DIRECTIONS:
-Lie on an incline, holding a pair of dumbbells at the sides of your lower chest with a neutral grip (palms facing each other).
-Squeeze your shoulder blades down and together and arch your lower back.
-Press the weights straight up until your arms are extended with a slight bend in the elbows.
-Pause for a moment at the top, then lower back to the sides of your lower chest. Repeat for reps.

TIP:
To avoid injury, place the dumbbells on your thighs and then move them to the floor when you finish your set.

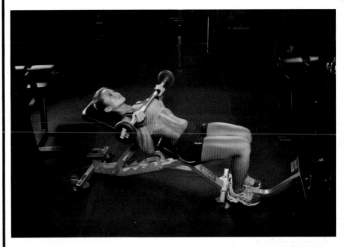

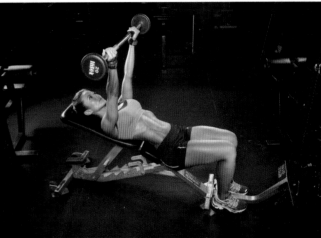

REVERSE-GRIP INCLINE PRESS
FOCUS AREA: UPPER CHEST, TRICEPS

ON THE FLIP SIDE: Unlike the overhand grip (which targets the mid-to-lower chest), the reverse grip (palms facing in) emphasizes the upper portion of the muscle—ideal if you're looking to give your cleavage a little boost.

DIRECTIONS:
-Lie faceup on an incline bench with your feet flat on the floor.
-Grasp the bar with a shoulder-width reverse grip (palms facing up).
-Lift the bar from the rack and fully extend your arms so that the bar is above your chest.
-Slowly lower the bar toward your lower chest, keeping your elbows pointed forward (not out to the sides).
-Pause, then press the bar toward the ceiling in a slight arc using a smooth, controlled motion.
-Stop just short of locking out your elbows. Repeat for reps.

TIP:
Perform this exercise using a spotter until you get used to the movement.

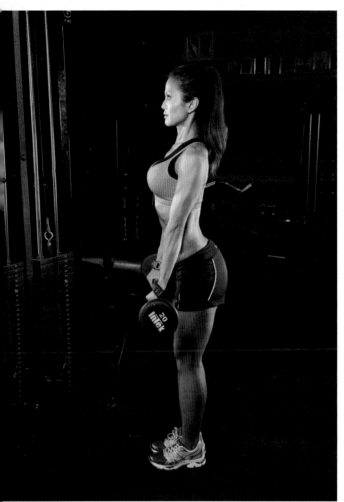
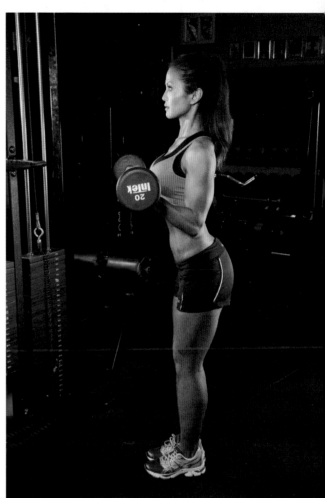

BICEPS

REVERSE-GRIP BARBELL CURL
FOCUS AREA: BRACHIALIS, UPPER FOREARM
ON THE FLIP SIDE: Shapely arms, they're not just for guys like Popeye anymore. By switching your grip to palms facing down, you place more focus on the biceps brachialis (side of the arm between the biceps and triceps) as well as your upper forearm. Using this move, you'll add more overall size and thickness to your biceps.

DIRECTIONS:
-Stand holding a barbell with an overhand grip.
-Keep your abs tight, chest up, and head straight.
-Contract your biceps to curl the bar toward your chest.
-Hold and squeeze at the top, then return the bar to the start. Repeat for reps.

TIP:
Wrap your thumbs around the bar for safety.

SAMPLE BICEPS WORKOUT

EXERCISE	SETS	REPS
Reverse-grip Barbell Curl*	5	15, 15, 12, 10,
Incline Dumbbell Curl	4	10
Reverse-grip Preacher Curl	3	10–12

*Includes two warmup sets of 15 reps each. Followin, warmup sets, working sets are performed pyramidin up in weight.

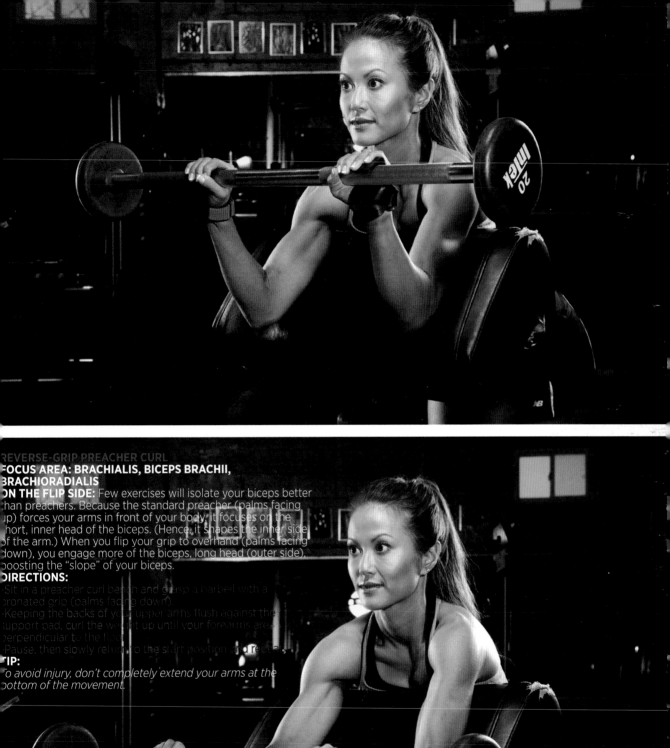

REVERSE-GRIP PREACHER CURL

FOCUS AREA: BRACHIALIS, BICEPS BRACHII, BRACHIORADIALIS

ON THE FLIP SIDE: Few exercises will isolate your biceps better than preachers. Because the standard preacher (palms facing up) forces your arms in front of your body, it focuses on the short, inner head of the biceps. (Hence, it shapes the inner side of the arm.) When you flip your grip to overhand (palms facing down), you engage more of the biceps, long head (outer side), boosting the "slope" of your biceps.

DIRECTIONS:
- Sit in a preacher curl bench and grasp a barbell with a pronated grip (palms facing down).
- Keeping the backs of your upper arms flush against the support pad, curl the weight up until your forearms are perpendicular to the floor.
- Pause, then slowly return to the start position and repeat.

TIP:
To avoid injury, don't completely extend your arms at the bottom of the movement.

SHOULDERS

**BARBELL REVERSE-GRIP
SHOULDER PRESS
FOCUS AREA: FRONT DELTS**
ON THE FLIP SIDE: If you're fighting flab under the arm, first you'll flip, then hit the chest-delt tie-in (the groove where the front delt meets the chest). Unlike the overhand grip version, the reverse grip (palms facing in) forces your elbows out in front of your body. This shifts the focus from the middle head of the delt to your front delts while also working the upper chest.
DIRECTIONS:
-Sit on a bench that adjusts to 90 degrees.
-Using an underhand, slightly wider than shoulder-width grip, start with the bar under your chin and just above your chest.
-Press the bar straight up until your arms are fully extended.
-Slowly lower the bar back to the start position and repeat.

SAMPLE SHOULDER WORKOUT

EXERCISE	SETS	REPS
Barbell Reverse-grip Shoulder Press	5	15, 15, 12, 10, 8
Cable Front Raises	2	12–15
Lateral Raises	3–4	8–10
Reverse Pec Deck	3	8–10

Includes two warmup sets of 15 reps each, followed by sets that pyramid up in weight.

**ALTERNATE EXERCISE:
DUMBBELL REVERSE-GRIP
SHOULDER PRESS**
-Sit squarely on a flat bench, shoulders back and chest up with your feet flat on the floor.
-Grasp a pair of dumbbells and raise your arms so that your hands line up with the tops of your ears, palms facing in.
-Press the weights straight up overhead until your arms are fully extended.
-Slowly lower the weight back to the start position and repeat.
TIP:
Don't bounce the weight back up at the bottom of the lift; use a slow, controlled motion.

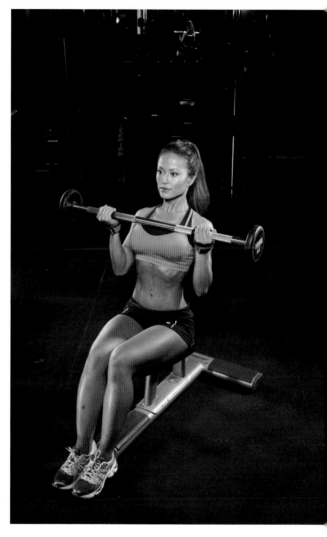

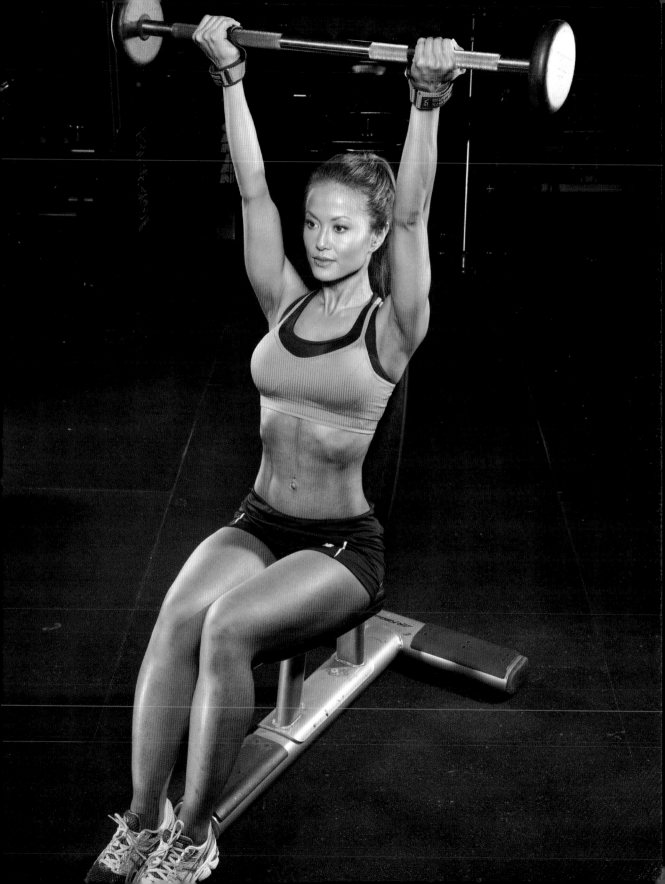

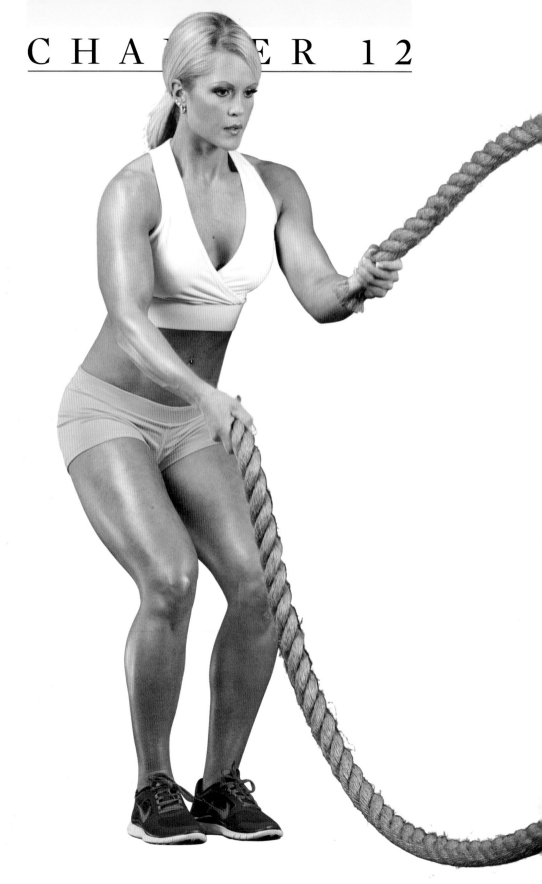

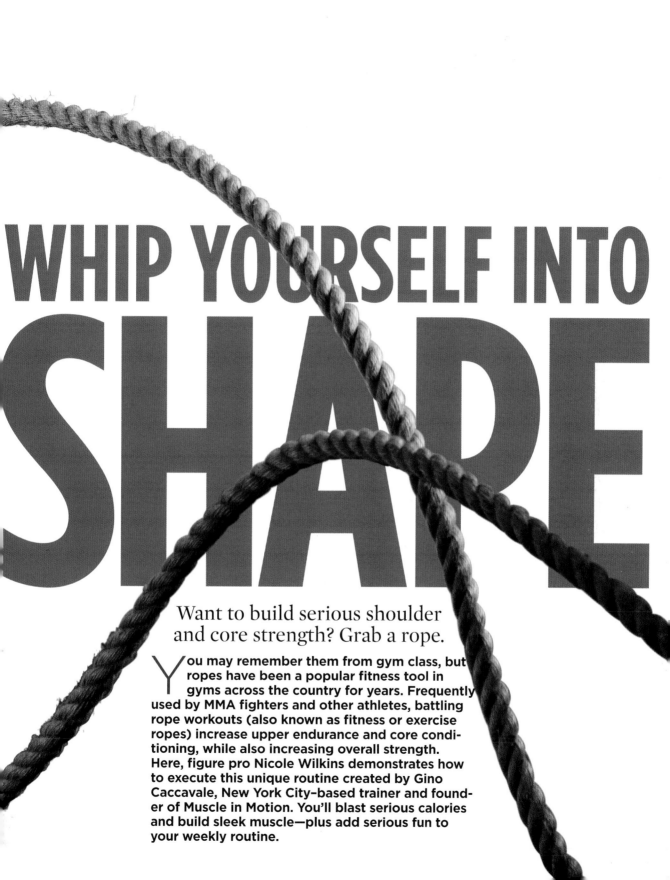

CHAPTER 12

WHIP YOURSELF INTO
SHAPE

Want to build serious shoulder
and core strength? Grab a rope.

Y ou may remember them from gym class, but
ropes have been a popular fitness tool in
gyms across the country for years. Frequently
used by MMA fighters and other athletes, battling
rope workouts (also known as fitness or exercise
ropes) increase upper endurance and core conditioning, while also increasing overall strength.
Here, figure pro Nicole Wilkins demonstrates how
to execute this unique routine created by Gino
Caccavale, New York City–based trainer and found-
er of Muscle in Motion. You'll blast serious calories
and build sleek muscle—plus add serious fun to
your weekly routine.

GETTING STARTED

For this workout you will need a set of battling ropes. Almost every commercial gym has a set of these now. If you want to purchase them, 50-foot ropes that are 1½ to two inches thick are the most common choice. Wear nonrestrictive workout clothes and training shoes that you feel grounded in, but that also have enough support to do some jumping.

Rope Climb

Works: Shoulders, Back, Arms, Core

This upper-body exercise not only works the arms but also requires an engaged core in order to help develop agility and coordination in your back.

>Reach your right hand above head level and grip the rope. Place left hand 12 inches below right. Bend your knees and wrap your right ankle and left heel around the bottom of the rope.

>Simultaneously drive your elbows down while pushing with your legs to lift off the floor. Remove your left hand from the rope and place it 12 inches above your right, and pull your body upward. Perform two sets of 20 pulls. To descend, reverse your arm movements while keeping your legs relaxed.

TIP

Don't just pull yourself up with your upper body and arms. Concentrate on pushing off with your legs as you move up the rope.

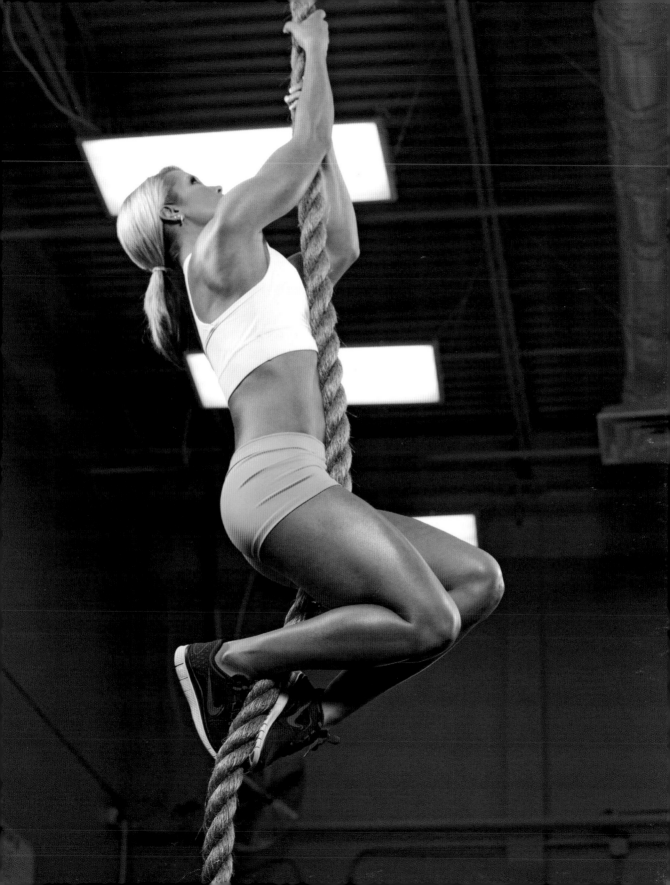

Double Rope Pullup

Works: Shoulders, Back, Arms, Core

This exercise focuses on your lats and can help improve functional fitness and increase muscle mass.

>Begin standing. Reach up and grab the two ropes, one in each hand. Pull your body upward while pushing elbows downward until your chin reaches hand level. Bend knees and cross ankles to create ground clearance as you lift off of the floor.

>Descend to almost a full hang, tapping toes lightly on the floor, then pull up again. Repeat two sets of 8–12 reps.

TIP

If it's too difficult to pull your body weight, jump into 90-degree arm position and hold.

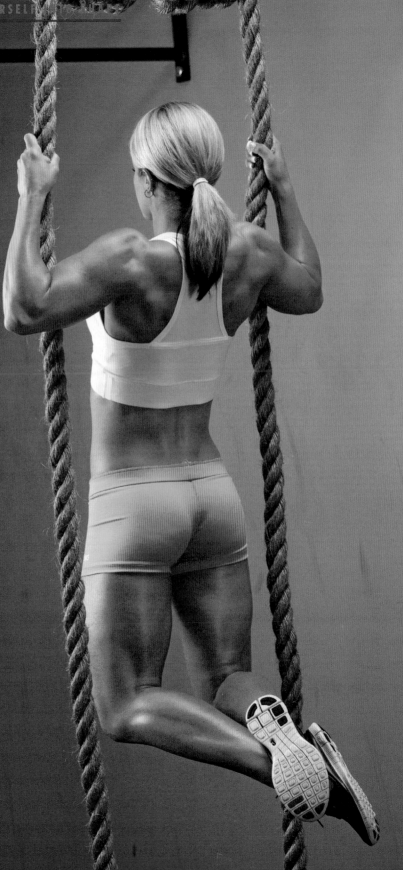

Cross-Arm Wave

Works: Shoulders, Back, Rear Delts, Core

The outward arm movement works your rear delts, which can help your posture.

>Start with your feet slightly parted, knees bent, core engaged. Grab ropes at hip level. Cross your left wrist and the rope over right wrist and rope, keeping elbows slightly bent. Pull ropes outward and back, pulling shoulder blades together.

>Return to start now with left wrist under right. Continue outward wave. Perform two sets, for one minute each.

TIP

Be sure to squeeze your shoulder blades together each time you move your arms outward.

Lateral Step Alternating Wave

Works: Shoulders, Core, Inner and Outer Thighs

This full-body exercise requires continuous movement of your arms and legs without pausing.

>Start with feet wider than hip width, knees bent, core engaged. Hold ropes at hip level. Keeping elbows bent, raise left arm to hip level.

>Push your right arm back down while simultaneously lifting your left arm to eye level. Continue waves.

>While doing waves, step your left foot to right. Return left foot to original squat position. Repeat with right foot. Do two sets for one minute.

TIP
Keep knees bent during sidestep without standing upright, to keep core engaged.

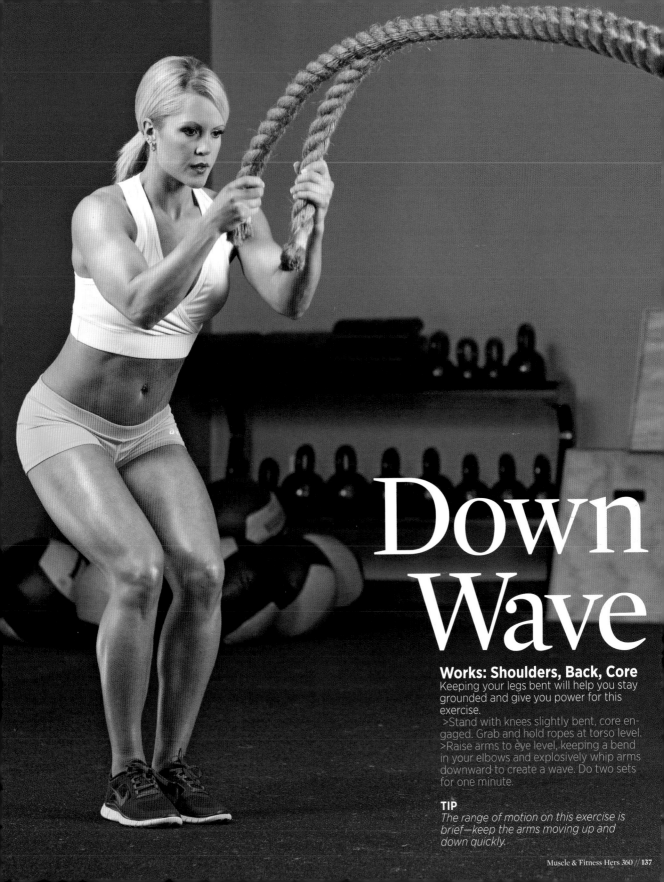

Down Wave

Works: Shoulders, Back, Core

Keeping your legs bent will help you stay grounded and give you power for this exercise.
>Stand with knees slightly bent, core engaged. Grab and hold ropes at torso level.
>Raise arms to eye level, keeping a bend in your elbows and explosively whip arms downward to create a wave. Do two sets for one minute.

TIP

The range of motion on this exercise is brief—keep the arms moving up and down quickly.

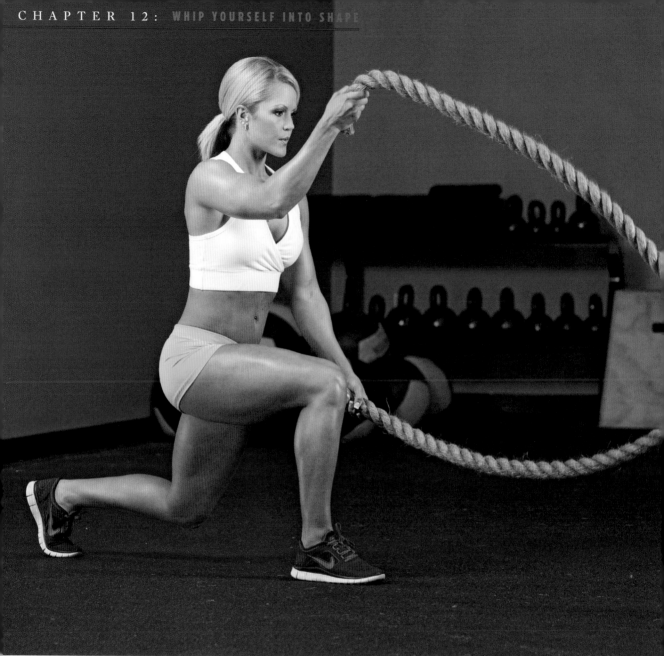

Alternating Two-Arm Lunging Wave

Works: Shoulders, Core, Legs

This move works the entire body and requires concentration on each muscle group.
>Stand with your knees bent, abs engaged. Hold ropes at hip level. Perform down waves, alternating your arms.
>At the same time, lunge left leg to the rear. Return to original quarter-squat position and repeat lunge back with right leg while still moving ropes. Perform two sets for one minute each.

TIP

Make sure you never lock your legs. It will make it difficult to engage your core.

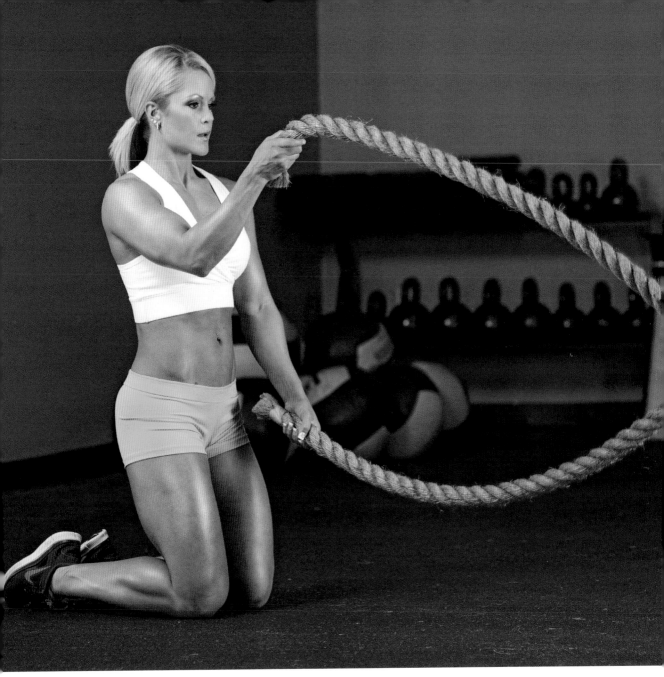

Kneeling Alt Wave

Works: Shoulders, Arms, Core

An engaged core and neutral spine are a must for this exercise.

>Kneel with knees six inches apart, core engaged. Hold ropes at hip level. Keeping elbows bent, raise right arm to eye level.

>Snap right arm to hip level while simultaneously lifting left arm to eye level. Repeat, creating a wave-like effect. Perform two sets for one minute each.

TIP

Keep your torso and thighs vertical throughout; don't lean back as you get tired.

Rope Jacks

Works: Shoulders, Core, Inner and Outer Thighs

The added cardio in this move really boo your calorie burn.

>Start with your feet together, holding a rope in each hand at your sides
>Jump feet outward like a standard jumping jack; raise arms and ropes overhead form a Y. Return to start; do two sets for one minute.

TIP

Do not lock your knees; keep them soft o both inward and outward leg movements

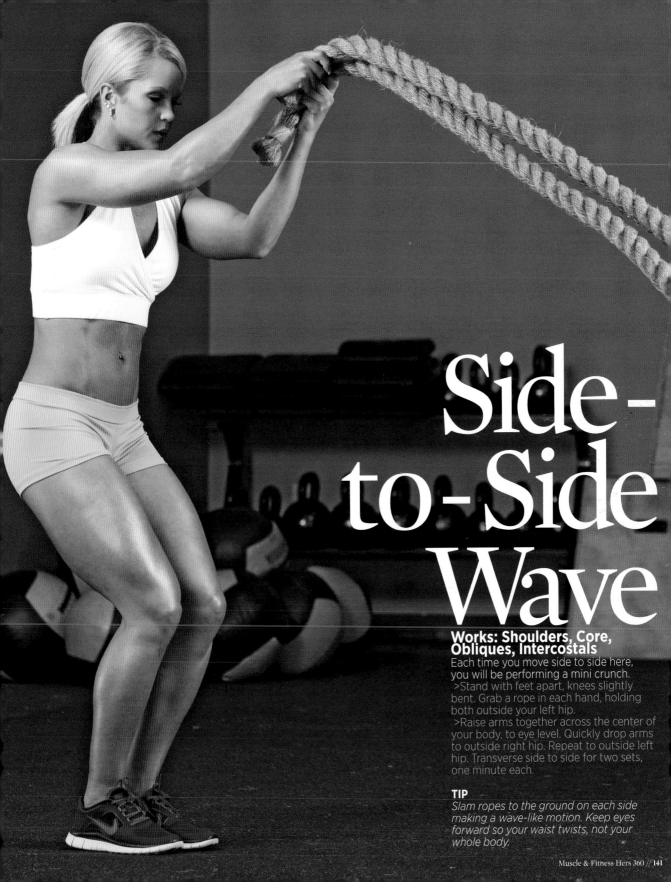

Side-to-Side Wave

Works: Shoulders, Core, Obliques, Intercostals

Each time you move side to side here, you will be performing a mini crunch.

>Stand with feet apart, knees slightly bent. Grab a rope in each hand, holding both outside your left hip.

>Raise arms together across the center of your body, to eye level. Quickly drop arms to outside right hip. Repeat to outside left hip. Transverse side to side for two sets, one minute each.

TIP

Slam ropes to the ground on each side making a wave-like motion. Keep eyes forward so your waist twists, not your whole body.

GET SHORT-CIRCUIT
SEXY

t's time for gorgeous, flawless muscle! Sculpting a bangin' body that'll inspire double-takes is faster than ever with interval-based Tabata-style training. Figure Olympia Pro Erin Stern does circuits of body-weight blasters and classic Olympic lifts to elevate her body to full-on fabulous, just 20 seconds at a time.

BODY-WEIGHT CIRCUIT

>Speed Squat >Dynamic Step-up >Speed Skater >Lunge Jump
Do each move at maximum effort for 20 sec.
Rest: 10 sec. between each move and 10 sec.
after each circuit.
Perform circuit twice.

OLYMPIC-LIFT CIRCUIT*

>Speed Squat >Dynamic Step-up >Speed Skater
Choose a weight that will max you out at 20 sec. If after 20 sec.
you could still do more, increase the weight. And if you can't
complete the move for 20 sec., go lighter.
Rest: 10 sec. between moves and 10 sec. between circuits.
Complete the circuit twice.
*Hold onto the Olympic bar for the entire circuit,
even during rest periods.

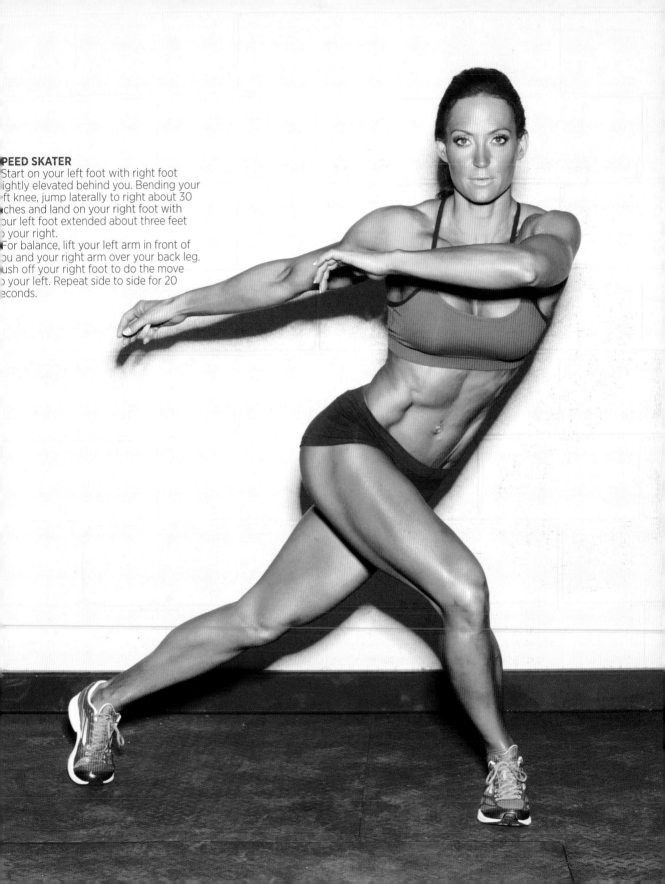

SPEED SKATER
Start on your left foot with right foot
lightly elevated behind you. Bending your
left knee, jump laterally to right about 30
inches and land on your right foot with
your left foot extended about three feet
to your right.
For balance, lift your left arm in front of
you and your right arm over your back leg.
Push off your right foot to do the move
to your left. Repeat side to side for 20
seconds.

SPEED SQUAT
>Stand in front of a low bench with your feet shoulder width and arms behind your head.
>Squat down quickly, until you make contact with the bench and then explosively return to the upright position. Do as many squats as you can for 20 seconds.

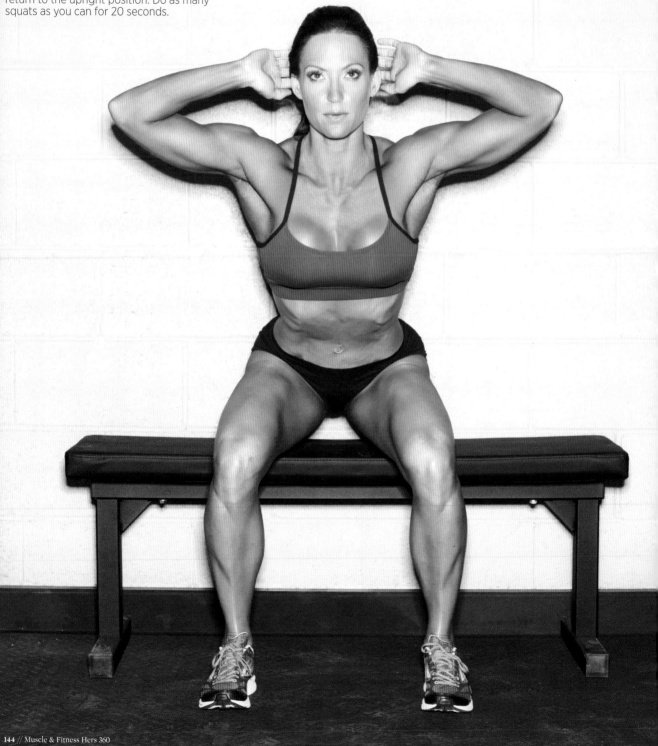

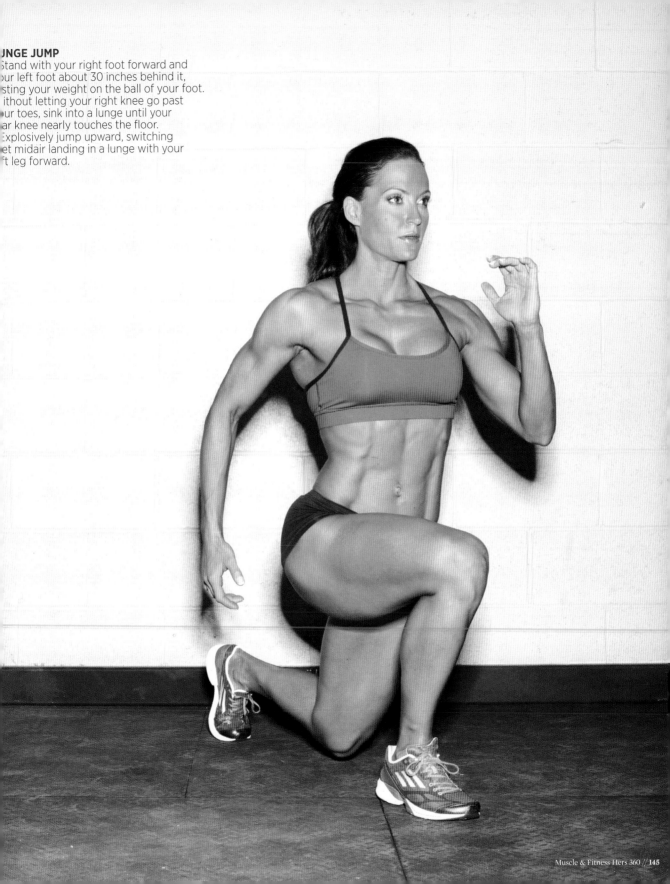

Stand with your right foot forward and
our left foot about 30 inches behind it,
sting your weight on the ball of your foot.
ithout letting your right knee go past
ur toes, sink into a lunge until your
ar knee nearly touches the floor.
Explosively jump upward, switching
et midair landing in a lunge with your
t leg forward.

ALTERNATING DYNAMIC STEP-UP
>Place right foot on an 18-inch box or bench. Explosively step onto the bench and swing your left knee toward your chest, letting your right foot leave the bench.
>Land on the bench on your left leg, then return your right leg to the floor. Pump your arms in a running motion for rhythm and stability. Alternate sides with each rep, doing as many reps as possible in 20 seconds.

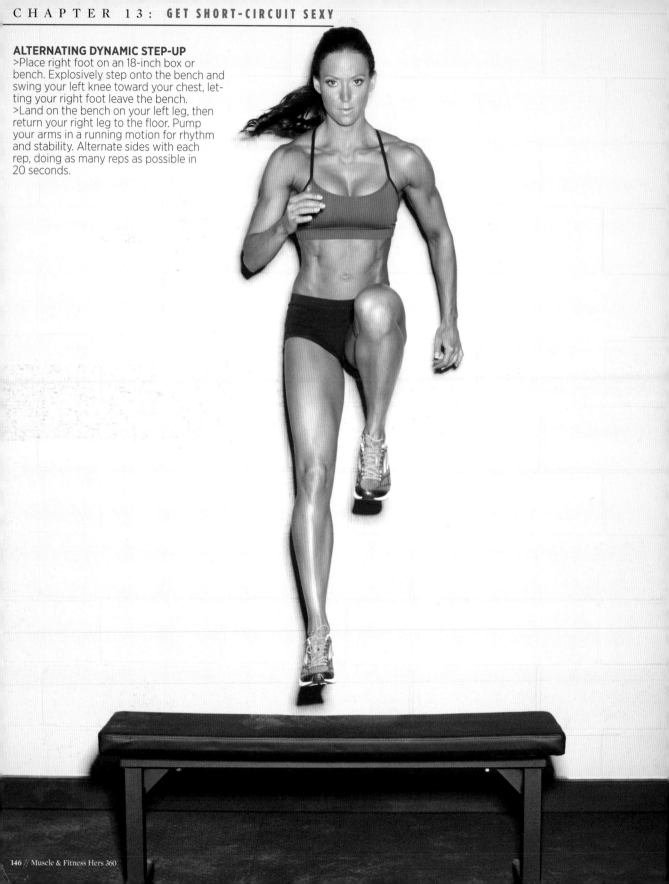

ROMANIAN DEADLIFT

Stand with feet hip width holding an Olympic bar in front of your thighs, hands shoulder width. Keeping your legs straight but without locking your knees, lower bar between your ankles and knees. Push off your heels to return to start. Repeat for max reps for 20 seconds.

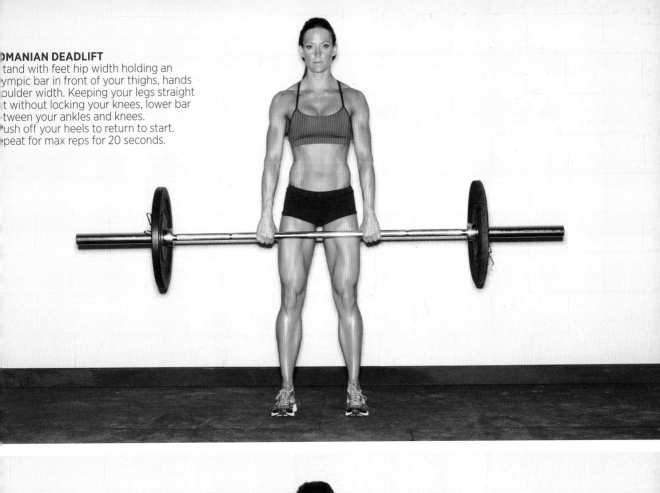

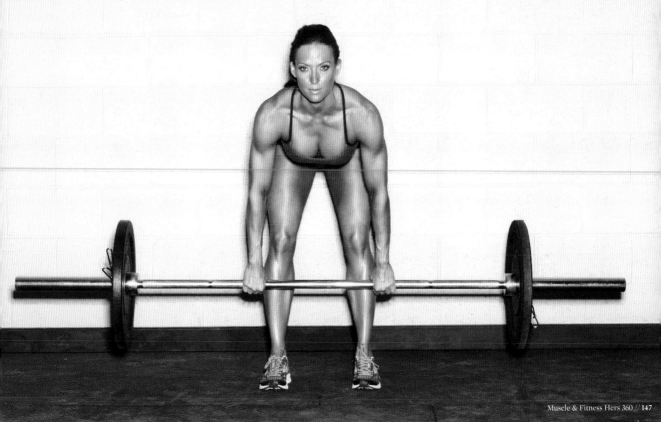

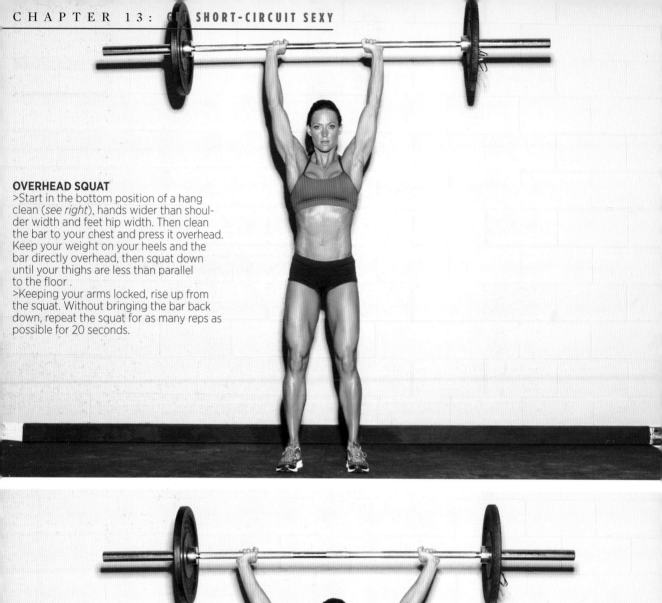

OVERHEAD SQUAT
>Start in the bottom position of a hang clean (*see right*), hands wider than shoulder width and feet hip width. Then clean the bar to your chest and press it overhead. Keep your weight on your heels and the bar directly overhead, then squat down until your thighs are less than parallel to the floor .
>Keeping your arms locked, rise up from the squat. Without bringing the bar back down, repeat the squat for as many reps as possible for 20 seconds.

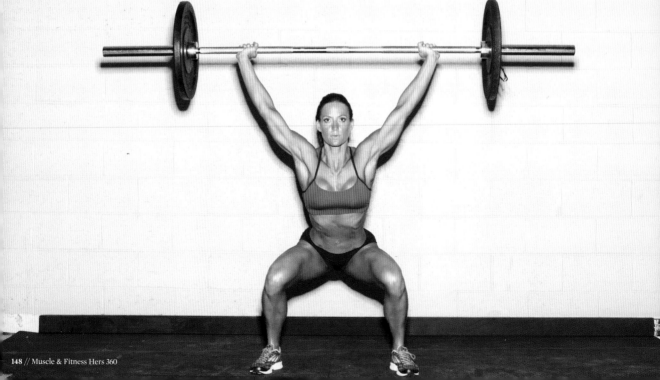

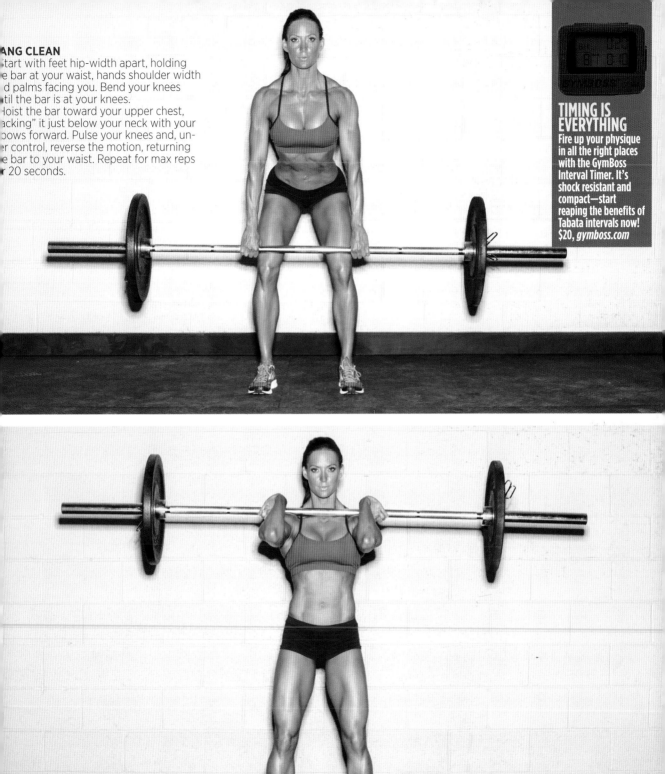

ANG CLEAN

Start with feet hip-width apart, holding
the bar at your waist, hands shoulder width
and palms facing you. Bend your knees
until the bar is at your knees.
Hoist the bar toward your upper chest,
"racking" it just below your neck with your
elbows forward. Pulse your knees and, under control, reverse the motion, returning
the bar to your waist. Repeat for max reps
for 20 seconds.

CHAPTER 14

NUTRITION 101

M&F Hers ultimate guide to eating right for the body you want

We don't want to burst your bubble, but a good, consistent training program alone won't even get you halfway to the body you want. Of course it's entirely necessary, and without one you won't reach your goals, but anyone who has been there and done that will tell you that the single most important factor in building the body you want is a proper nutrition plan. Here, we've compiled a user-friendly, comprehensive nutrition guide that addresses all of your most pressing food-related questions. Get going and get ready for your best body ever!

QUICK TIP A weight-loss calorie intake level for most active women would be about 12 calories per pound of body weight daily.

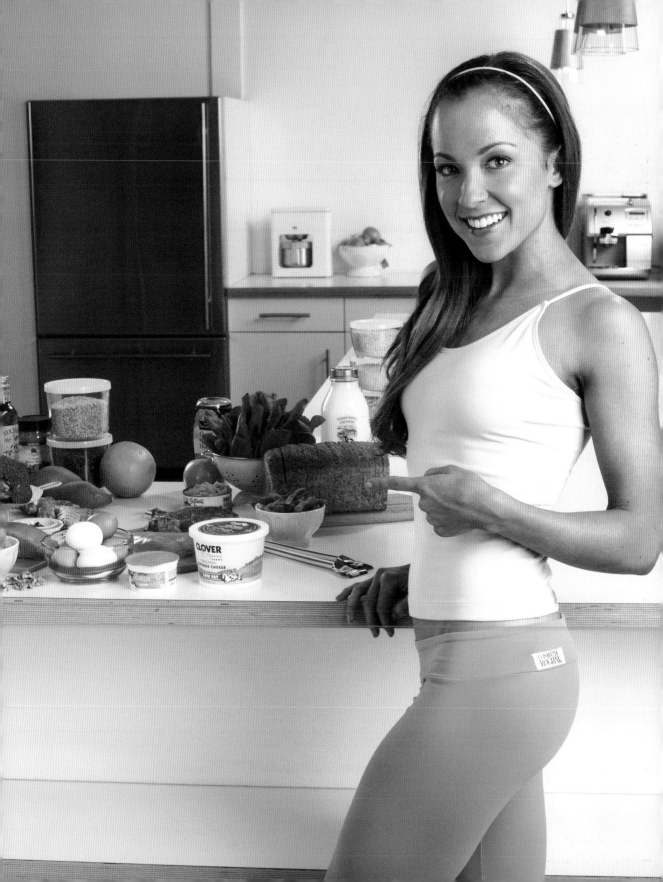

NUTRITION Q&A

Everything you ever wanted to know about nutrition for fit chicks

1 **If weight loss (and maintenance) really comes down to the matter of calories in versus calories out, can I reach my goal by staying under a certain amount of calories per day?**
True, the most important factor for weight loss is burning more calories than you eat. But to ensure you're burning off body fat and not muscle—and to build muscle while burning body fat—your macronutrient intake becomes critical. Since muscle is composed of protein, it makes sense that you need ample amounts of protein. So when trying to drop body fat, you don't want to lower protein intake.

We now know that eating fat does not lead to fat gain, especially when you eat the right kinds—namely, essential fats like the omega-3 and monounsaturated fats. In fact, these fats actually encourage fat loss.

Unlike protein and fat, which are essential, there are no essential carbs. That's because your body can convert protein and fat into carbs. So to lose fat you should start by reducing carb intake. This method also helps to keep insulin levels low and steady, which allows for greater fat burning and less fat gain.

2 **What combination of macronutrients should a healthy, active woman shoot for on a daily basis?**
Typically we suggest about 1 to 1.5g of protein, about 1 g of carbs or less, and about 0.25 to 0.5g of fat per pound of body weight. That comes out to about 11–15 calories per pound of body weight.

3 **Aside from protein, carbs, and fat, what should I be looking at on nutrition labels as far as what to eat and what to avoid?**
Most of the food you eat should be fresh, unpackaged food that doesn't necessarily have a nutrition label on it—fish, chicken, steak, eggs, veggies, and fruit. This—along with your supplements—is where your micronutrients, such as vitamins and minerals, will be coming from. With packaged foods, focus on the major macros. Fiber is part of the carb macro, so the more fiber the better. And check that the sugar content is less than half the total carbs. Also be sure that there are zero trans fats, as well as nothing "hydrogenated" or "partially hydrogenated"—code words for trans fats.

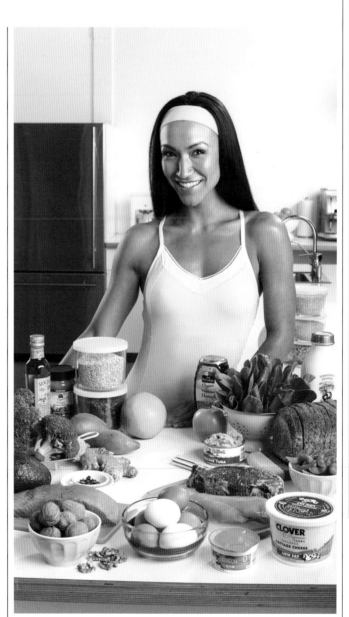

4 **If weight loss is predominantly about calories in versus calories out, isn't it better to skip meals if I'm not hungry?**
Not really, as that can put your body into starvation mode, which slows your metabolism down and causes you to store more fat when you do eat.

THE GLYCEMIC INDEX

The glycemic index (GI) ranks carbohydrates according to their effect on blood sugar levels. Low GI foods are burned steadily throughout the day to give you a constant supply of energy. High GI foods are readily transported to fat cells if you don't burn them off quickly.

Choosing low GI carbs, the ones that produce only small fluctuations in blood glucose and insulin levels—is the secret to long-term health and reducing your risk of heart disease and diabetes, and is the key to sustainable weight loss. *Hers* recommends high-GI foods only after training to spike insulin levels in order to spark lean muscle growth.

GI CHART

Foods in the low category usually have GI values of 55 or less; in the medium category, a GI value of 56–69; and in the high category, a GI of 70 or more.

BROCCOLI
GRAPEFRUIT
APPLE
WHOLE-GRAIN BREAD
SWEET POTATO
OATMEAL
PIZZA, CHEESE
SPAGHETTI
WHITE RICE
TABLE SUGAR (SUCROSE)
WHITE BREAD
WATERMELON
RICE CAKES (WHITE)
JELLY BEANS
WHITE POTATO (BAKED)

OMEGA-3 FATTY ACIDS
can be found in fish such
as salmon, tuna, and
halibut; some plants;
and nut oils.

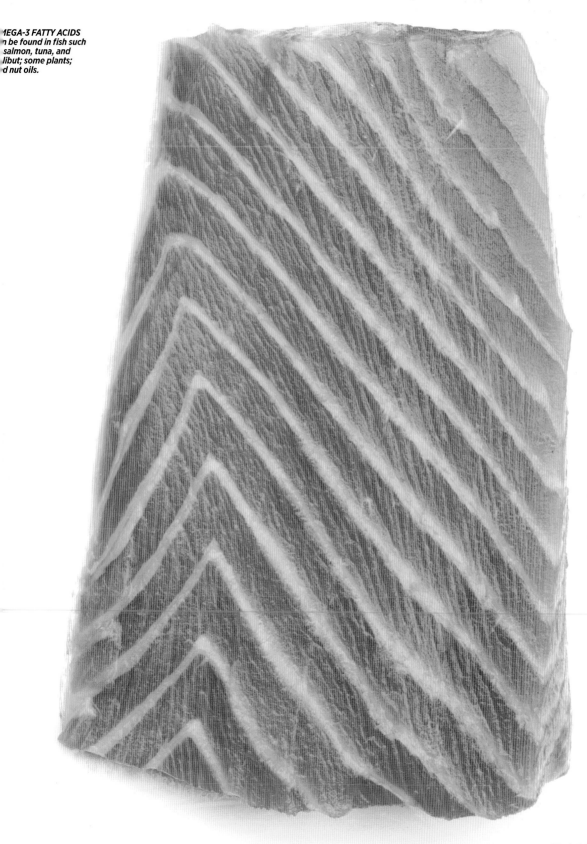

CARBS DEFINED

A predominant energy source for your body, carbohydrates are found in a wide range of foods, such as pasta, grains, fruits, and veggies. During digestion, carbohydrate molecules are absorbed into the bloodstream and shuttled to individual cells. There, glucose—the most common form of carbohydrate—is transformed into glycogen for later use or used directly for energy. Once the body's glycogen stores are full, any extra carbohydrate is synthesized into fat.

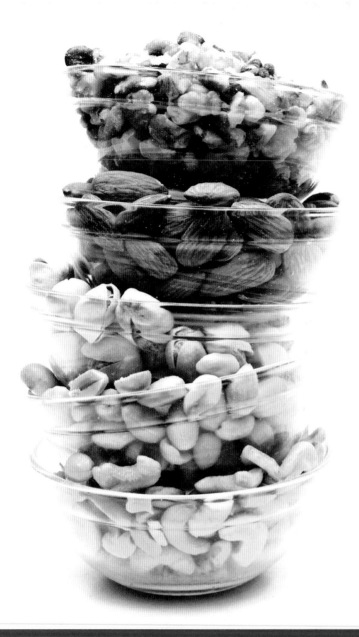

5 **What are the pros and cons of low-carb diets?**
A lot of people complain they have no energy when eating low carb and have difficulty working out. This is true during the first couple of weeks on a low-carb diet. That's because in those who have been eating higher carbs, their bodies have adapted to burning carbs as a primary fuel source. When those ample carbs are suddenly gone, the body first struggles to burn adequate amounts of fat for fuel. However, after a few weeks of sticking with a low-carb diet, the body adapts by increasing the enzymes involved in burning fat, and becomes more efficient at burning fat for fuel.

6 **Can I stay on a low-carb diet forever?**
One problem with low-carb and low-calorie diets is that if you stay on them for too long, your leptin levels will drop. Since leptin keeps your metabolic rate up and your hunger down, lower levels mean that your metabolic rate also drops and your hunger rises. To prevent this, those on a very low-carb plan (less than 0.5g per pound) should have a high-carb (2g or more per pound), high-calorie day once per week.

7 **Can a low-carb diet be maintained year-round, even after I've reached my goal?**
Yes, there really is no reason to go back to a high-carb diet for prolonged periods. However, as stated in No. 6, when you follow a very low-carb and low-calorie diet, your levels of the hormone leptin can start to decline. So just make sure to keep up the weekly high-carb, high-calorie day. But, for long-term health and fitness, *Hers* editors generally recommend a balanced ratio of macronutrients (protein, carbs, fat) somewhere closer to equal amounts, 40/30/30, for example.

8 **What are the best and worst sources of carbs?**
Obviously, you want to focus on slow-digesting carbs at most meals—oatmeal, sweet potatoes, whole grains, and some fruit. One really problematic carb is fructose, which is found in fruit and in products using high-fructose corn syrup. Fructose is a sugar the body doesn't use well. The majority of fructose we consume gets converted to glucose in the body, mainly in the liver. But when there are ample glucose stores, the liver converts fructose into fat. So it's hard to predict whether that piece of fruit is going to be stored as glycogen or converted into fat.

KNOW YOUR FATS
THE GOOD

>Monounsaturated fats lower total cholesterol and LDL cholesterol (the bad cholesterol) while increasing HDL cholesterol (the good cholesterol). Nuts (walnuts, almonds), avocados, and canola and olive oil are high in MUFAs. MUFAs have also been found to help in weight loss, particularly of body fat.

>Polyunsaturated fats also lower total cholesterol and LDL cholesterol. Seafood like salmon and fish oil, as well as corn, soy, safflower, and sunflower oils are high in polyunsaturated fats. Omega-3 fatty acids belong to this group.

THE BAD

>Saturated fats raise total blood cholesterol as well as LDL cholesterol. Saturated fats are mainly found in animal products such as meat, dairy, eggs, and seafood. Some plant foods, such as coconut oil, palm oil, and palm kernel oil are also high in saturated fats.

>Trans fats were invented when scientists began to "hydrogenate" liquid oils so that they could better withstand the food-production process and give foods a longer shelf life. As a result of hydrogenation, trans fatty acids are formed. Trans fatty acids are found in many commercially packaged foods, in commercially fried food such as French fries from some fast-food chains, and in other packaged snacks such as microwave popcorn, as well as in vegetable shortening and hard-stick margarine.

CALORIE COUNTER
Calories per gram in the macronutrients
PROTEIN: 4 CAL/GRAM
CARBS: 4 CAL/GRAM
FAT: 9 CAL/GRAM

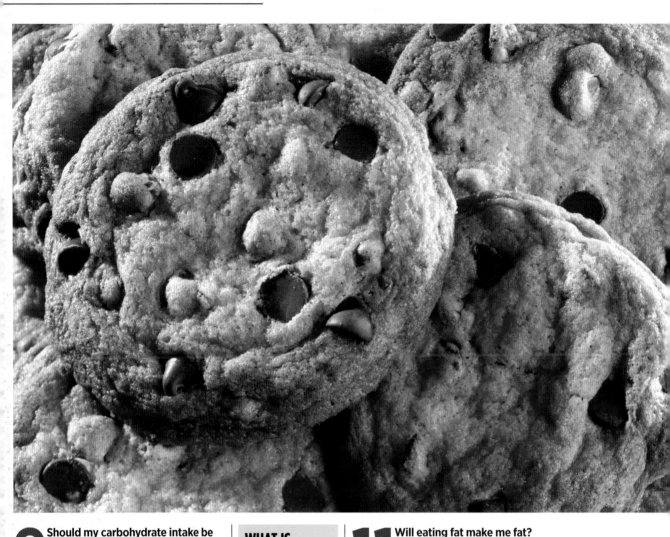

9 Should my carbohydrate intake be tapered throughout the day?

Yes, most women should taper carbs, because insulin sensitivity is lower later in the day. That means that you have to release more insulin for the same amount of carbs—and since insulin inhibits fat burning, that can be bad. If you train later in the evening, you don't need to curb your intake of carbs around workouts, however, since they will be used to fuel the workout and recovery and thus won't be stored as body fat.

10 Should I avoid dairy when trying to get lean?

Not necessarily. Dairy—especially organic dairy—is not only a very high-quality protein source that is rich in gluta-mine, but it is a good source of conjugated lin-oleic acid and omega-3 fats. (For more on this, see "The 15 Best Lean-Muscle-Building Foods" at the end of this chapter.) Whey protein and casein protein powders come from dairy. You simply can't get a better protein source around workouts, so why avoid them?

WHAT IS ORGANIC?

The United States Department of Agriculture (USDA) defines "organic" as foods that are produced without antibiotics, hormones, pesticides, irradiation, or bioengineering. Organic farmers are required to adhere to certain soil and water conservation methods and to rules about the humane treatment of animals.

11 Will eating fat make me fat?

Not if you are eating the right kind of fats. Fat is an energy source, just as carbs and protein are. But fats also perform important functions in the body. They are used to make up cell membranes, such as those that encase muscle cells. The essenti. fats—omega-3s and omega-6s—are used in the body to make critic. chemical messengers known as prostaglandins. These are importan for joint and muscle recovery, as well as numerous other important functions. Now we know that omega-3 fats also activate genes that encourage fat burning and blunt fat storage. You need about 20–30 percent of your total daily calories to come from fat.

12 What's the right way to cheat on a diet?

It is actually beneficial for those eating a low-carb diet to cheat once a week by having a very high-carb day (at least 2g of carbs per pound of body weight). For those c a moderate-carb, maintenance diet or who are trying to add muscle try a cheat meal once per week—anything you want, like pizza or a burger and fries. And dessert. Eat what you crave most. This one me won't derail your progress—it will help it, as mentioned in rule No. 6, and also make a world of difference in your sanity while dieting. Wh you allow yourself this one cheat meal per week, it's a carrot you car dangle in front of yourself. You are actually less likely to cheat the res of the week. After that cheat meal, most people feel satisfied and ready for another week of clean eating before cheating again.

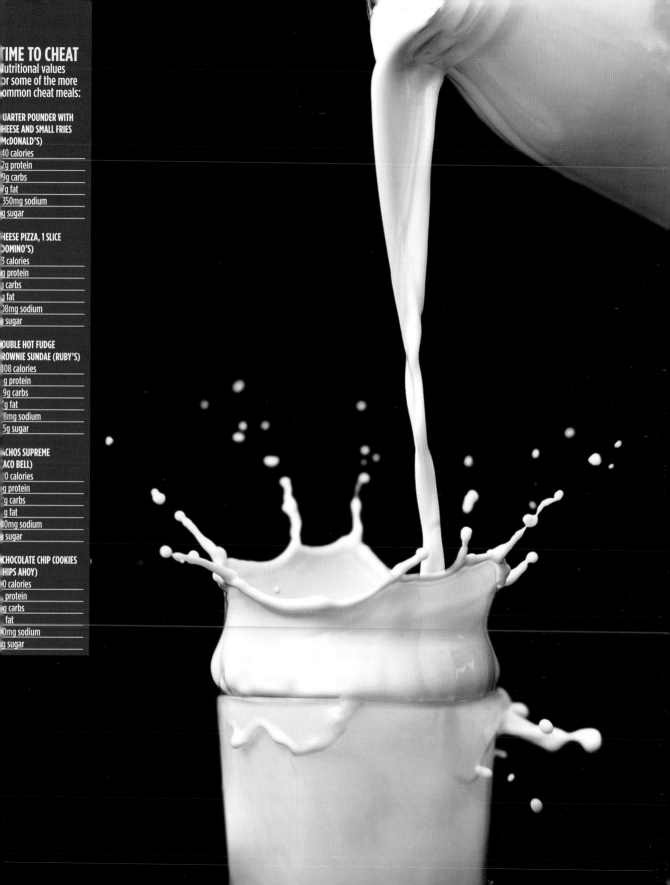

TIME TO CHEAT
Nutritional values
for some of the more
common cheat meals:

**QUARTER POUNDER WITH
CHEESE AND SMALL FRIES
(McDONALD'S)**
840 calories
42g protein
99g carbs
37g fat
1350mg sodium
9g sugar

**CHEESE PIZZA, 1 SLICE
(DOMINO'S)**
273 calories
9g protein
34g carbs
10g fat
508mg sodium
3g sugar

**DOUBLE HOT FUDGE
BROWNIE SUNDAE (RUBY'S)**
1108 calories
12g protein
149g carbs
47g fat
818mg sodium
115g sugar

**NACHOS SUPREME
(TACO BELL)**
440 calories
13g protein
38g carbs
26g fat
800mg sodium
4g sugar

**3 CHOCOLATE CHIP COOKIES
(CHIPS AHOY)**
160 calories
2g protein
22g carbs
8g fat
110mg sodium
11g sugar

TIPS TO CHOOSE YOUR BOOZE

• **RED WINE (5 oz):**
125 calories, 0g protein, 4g carbs, 0g fat (108 calories come from alcohol content) Low in calories due to low sugar content; contains resveratrol, a super-antioxidant that may help combat cancer and reduce signs of aging (among other benefits).

• **WHITE WINE (5 oz):**
121 calories, 0g protein, 4g carbs, 0g fat (105 calories come from alcohol content) Low in calories and carbs, but has less phenols and antioxidants than red wine. White wine is better than many alcohols, but red wine wins on all counts.

• **BEER (10 oz):**
126 calories, 2g protein, 10g carbs, 0g fat (76 calories come from alcohol content) Good for an antioxidant boost but with a lot of calories on the side. Light beers come closer to the carb content of white wine, and are the healthier choice.

• **MARGARITA (5 oz):**
230 calories, 0.5g protein, 10g carbs, 0g fat (189 calories come from alcohol content) A margarita is made with tequila, triple sec, lime juice, sugar, and ice and is usually served on the rocks. Not typically considered nutritious, the alcohol and sugar provide the calorie count and the lime juice proffers some vitamin C. Traditionally served in a salt-rimmed glass, the margarita is also high in sodium.

• **MOJITO (5 oz):**
215 calories, 0g protein, 8.5g carbs, 0g fat (179 calories come from alcohol content) Because the flavor, for the most part, comes from fresh mint and limes (and a teaspoon or two of sugar), the calorie count here is lighter than a cocktail mixed with flavored syrup.

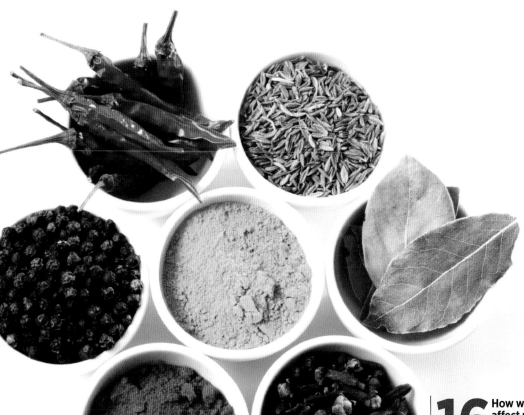

POST-WORK-OUT FUEL

For athletes, the best way to refuel your muscles and recover stronger is by consuming some fast-digesting carbs, such as sugar or better yet, pure dextrose, after a workout. Although you should avoid these foods most of the day, avoiding them after exercise actually hampers your progress.

16 How will drinking alcohol affect my diet?
Alcohol is not as bad as you may think, as long as you consume it in moderation. Research shows those who are moderate drinkers do not gain as much weight over the years as those who abstain. In fact, hard liquor and wine offer certain health benefits. Alcohol itself doesn't get converted into body fat; however, excessive alcohol can alter the biochemistry of the body to make fat storage easier. So try to keep it to a glass or two of alcohol once or twice per week.

17 Are some vegetables better than others?
All vegetables are good if you stick with true vegetables. True vegetables are low in starchy carbs but high in fiber. These include foods like broccoli, asparagus, spinach, kale, and cauliflower. Corn is high in starchy carbs, but it is technically not a veggie, even though most people think of it that way. Corn is actually a grain, much like wheat and rice. One cup of corn has over 40g of carbs, whereas one cup of chopped broccoli has only 6g. And, obviously, watch your intake of potatoes, which are classified as tubers. White potatoes are not only very starchy, but they digest very rapidly, which spikes insulin levels.

QUICK TIP
Choose darker salad greens such as red leaf and green leaf, which have more nutrients than lighter greens such as iceberg.

13 Do I need to weigh my food before each meal? What if I don't have a food scale?
You do not need to weigh all ...d. When you buy meat, the weight is on ...package. You can estimate the weight of ...hicken breast by dividing the number of ...cken breasts in the package by the total ...ght of the package. For other common ...ds, here's a helpful cheat sheet you can ... in lieu of a food scale:

ASURING STICK	FOOD
-cream scooper	½ cup cooked rice/pasta/oatmeal
nis ball	1 medium fruit (apple/orange/pear)
-yo	Bagel
t	4 oz chicken/beef/turkey/fish
umb	1 oz cheese
ndful	1 serving nuts (almonds/walnuts/cashews)

14 What are the best and worst condiments to use?
The worst condiments are those that contain high fructose corn syrup, as many ketchups and barbecue sauces do. Mustards are great, as the mustard seed has been shown to boost fat burning. And soy sauce is fine, too—in moderation—as it is low in calories.

15 Can I season my foods? Which seasonings are OK to use and which should I stay away from?
Yes, do yourself a favor and season your foods to enhance the flavor. It's easier to eat "clean" when the food tastes good. The absolute best seasonings and spices are cayenne pepper, garlic, and ginger, since these not only punch up the flavor of your foods, but also punch up your fat burning and provide numerous other health benefits. Salt is fine, too, as you only need to worry about cutting sodium during the final week before a contest or photo shoot.

GOAL: BURN FAT ONE-WEEK MEAL PLAN

The following plan is designed for a woman weighing 140 pounds. When trying to lose weight during a rigorous exercise program, shoot for an intake of about 12 calories per pound of body weight. So for a 110-pound woman, total daily calories would be approximately 1,320; for a 150-pound woman, about 1,800. Here, a few quick and tasty Burn Fat Meal Plan recipes.

A TURKEY ROLLS

4 slices turkey deli meat
2 slices reduced-fat swiss cheese (Alpine Lace)
Place two slices of turkey together and lay one slice of cheese on top; spread mustard on cheese and roll into a tube and eat.

B BREAKFAST BURRITO

1 large whole large egg
1 large egg white
1 slice reduced-fat American cheese
2 slices low-fat deli ham
10" whole-wheat pita
Heat tortilla in warm pan; fry ham in pan and place on tortilla; scramble eggs and cook in pan sprayed with nonstick cooking spray, add cheese and place on tortilla; roll tortilla into breakfast burrito.

C CHILI CON CARNE

6 oz lean ground beef (90% lean)
¼ can (14½ oz) diced tomatoes with chilies
¼ medium onion (diced)
½ tsp cumin
1 tsp red chili pepper flakes
Salt and pepper to taste
Brown beef in pan; add tomatoes and onion, cumin, chili pepper flakes, and salt and pepper to taste.

D OMELET

1 large whole egg
2 large egg whites
2 tbsp light cream cheese
½ cup raw spinach
Scramble the eggs in a pan with olive oil or nonfat cooking spray; flip eggs; mix together cream cheese and spinach in a bowl; spread cream cheese mixture onto cooked side of egg. Wait 30 seconds to ensure the other side of the egg is cooked, fold in half, wait 1 minute, until cream cheese mixture is melted.

E BREAKFAST PIZZA

1 large whole egg
¼ Boboli whole-wheat pizza crust
¼ cup fat-free mozzarel
2 slices Jennie-O extra lean turkey bacon
Beat egg in a bowl and drizzle half over the cru spread cheese over cru and drizzle the rest of t egg over the cheese; to with bacon; bake in ove at 450 degrees for 10 minutes or until egg is cooked and cheese is melted.

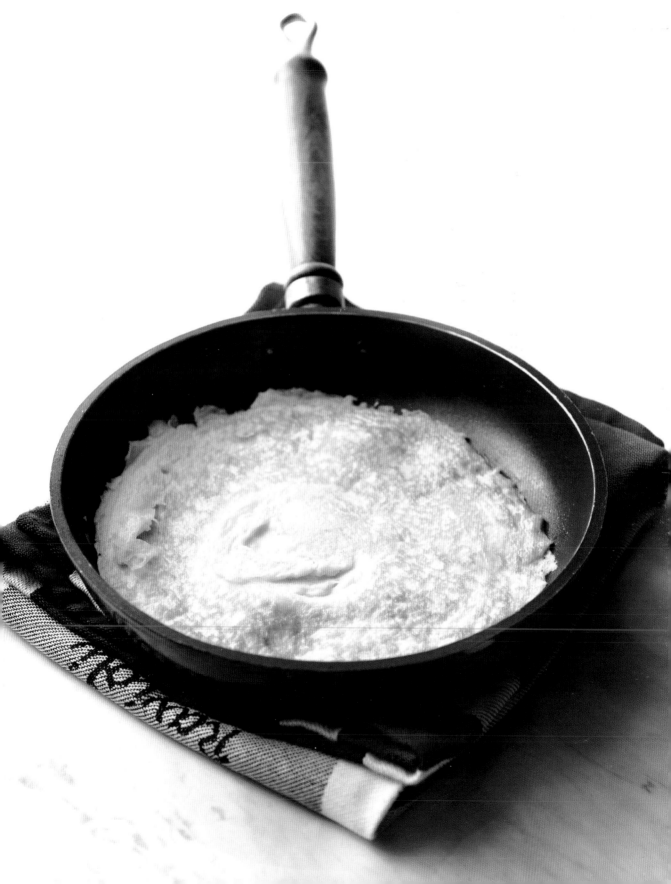

MONDAY

BREAKFAST 1
1 scoop whey protein
½ large grapefruit

BREAKFAST 2
(30–60 minutes after B1)
Western Bagel
Perfect 10 Healthy
Grain Bagel
1 tbsp peanut butter

LATE-MORNING SNACK
2 large whole eggs,
hard-boiled

LUNCH
Turkey Rolls
(Recipe A)

MIDDAY SNACK
3 oz albacore tuna,
in water
¼ cup low-fat
cottage cheese
*(Mix cottage cheese
in tuna; add any de-
sired vegetables.)*

DINNER
6 oz shrimp
1 cup frozen stir-fry
vegetables
¼ small ginger root,
thinly sliced
1 tbsp soy sauce
*(Stir-fry veggies and
shrimp, then add gin-
ger and soy sauce.)*
2 cups mixed green
salad *(include spin-
ach and raw broccoli)*
1 tbsp olive oil and
1 tbsp balsamic
vinegar *(use as salad
dressing.)*

NIGHTTIME SNACK
1 scoop casein
protein
7 walnut halves
Totals: 1,565 calories,
185g protein, 65g
carbs, 65g fat

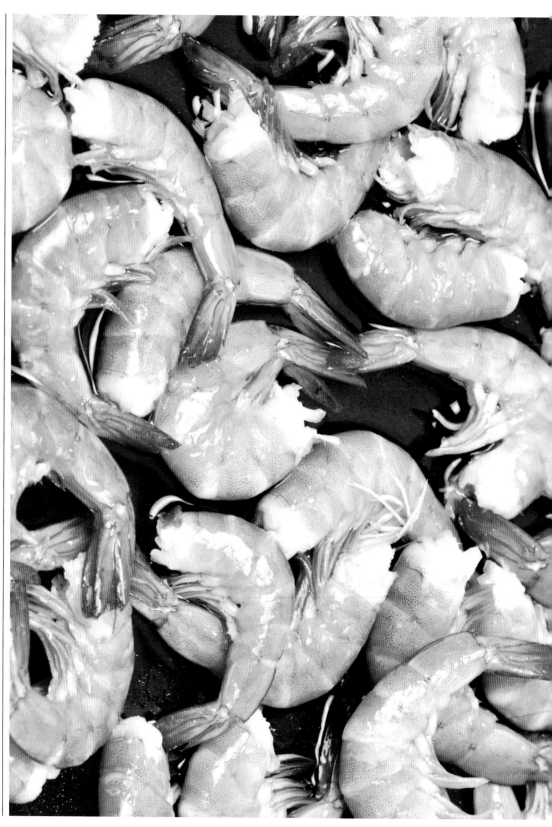

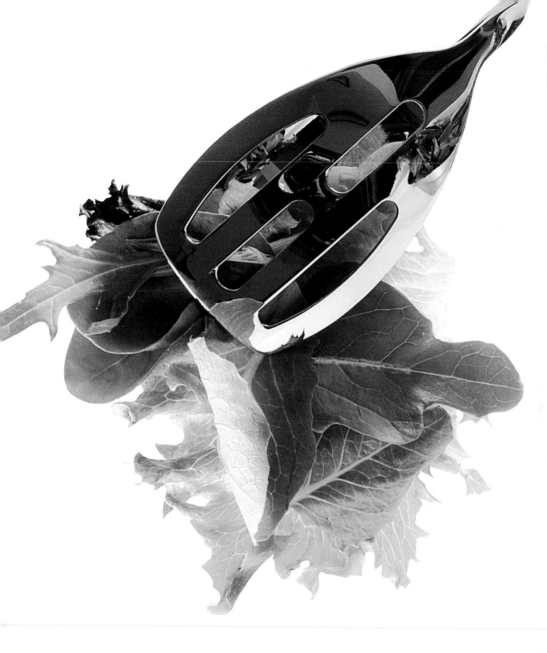

TUESDAY

BREAKFAST 1
1 scoop whey protein
½ large grapefruit

BREAKFAST 2
2 large whole eggs
3 slices Jennie-O extra-lean turkey bacon
1 cup cooked oatmeal

LATE-MORNING SNACK
½ cup cottage cheese

LUNCH
6 oz chicken breast
2 cups mixed green salad
1 tbsp olive oil and
1 tbsp balsamic vinegar *(use as salad dressing)*

MIDDAY SNACK
½ cup reduced-fat Greek yogurt
1 tbsp peanut butter
(Mix peanut butter in yogurt.)

DINNER
6 oz salmon
½ cup mixed frozen veggies
2 cups mixed green salad *(include spinach and raw broccoli)*
1 tbsp olive oil and
1 tbsp balsamic vinegar *(use as salad dressing)*

NIGHTTIME SNACK
½ cup cottage cheese
2 tbsp salsa
(Mix salsa in cottage cheese.)

Totals: 1,715 calories, 170g protein, 80g carbs, 75g fat

WEDNESDAY

BREAKFAST 1
1 scoop whey protein
½ large grapefruit

BREAKFAST 2
2 large whole eggs
1 whole egg white
⅛ cup fat-free cheddar cheese
(*Make a cheese omelet.*)
1 whole-grain waffle (*such as Van's*)
2 tbsp fat-free Reddi-Wip
(*Top waffle with whipped cream.*)

LATE-MORNING SNACK
1 scoop whey protein
1 tbsp peanut butter

LUNCH
3 oz albacore tuna, in water
2 cups mixed green salad (*include spinach and raw broccoli*)
1 tbsp olive oil and
1 tbsp balsamic vinegar (*use as salad dressing*)
(*Top salad with tuna.*)

MIDDAY SNACK
Turkey Rolls (Recipe A) **+ Avocado**
2 slices low-fat American cheese
2 slices low-fat deli ham
¼ avocado
(*Top a slice of ham with a slice of cheese. Place a slice of avocado in the middle and roll up. Repeat with the other slice of ham, cheese, and avocado.*)

DINNER
6 oz chicken breast
1 cup chopped broccoli
2 cups mixed green salad (*include spinach and raw broccoli*)
1 tbsp olive oil and
1 tbsp balsamic vinegar (*use as salad dressing*)

NIGHTTIME SNACK
1 scoop casein protein
Totals: 1,600 calories, 180g protein, 65g carbs, 65g fat

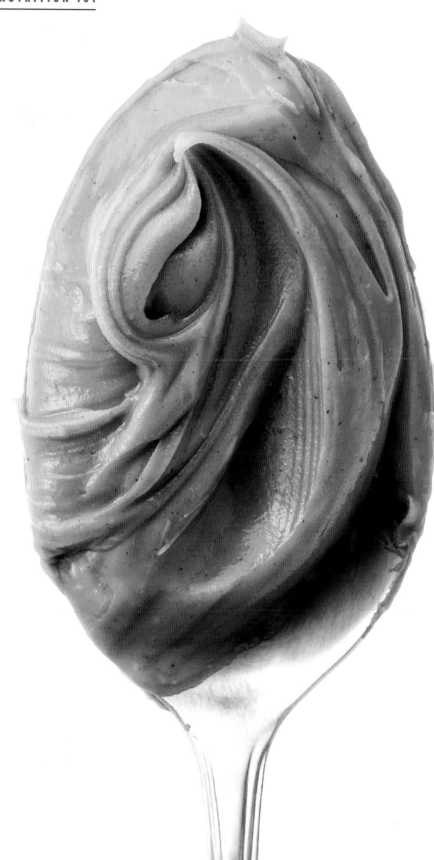

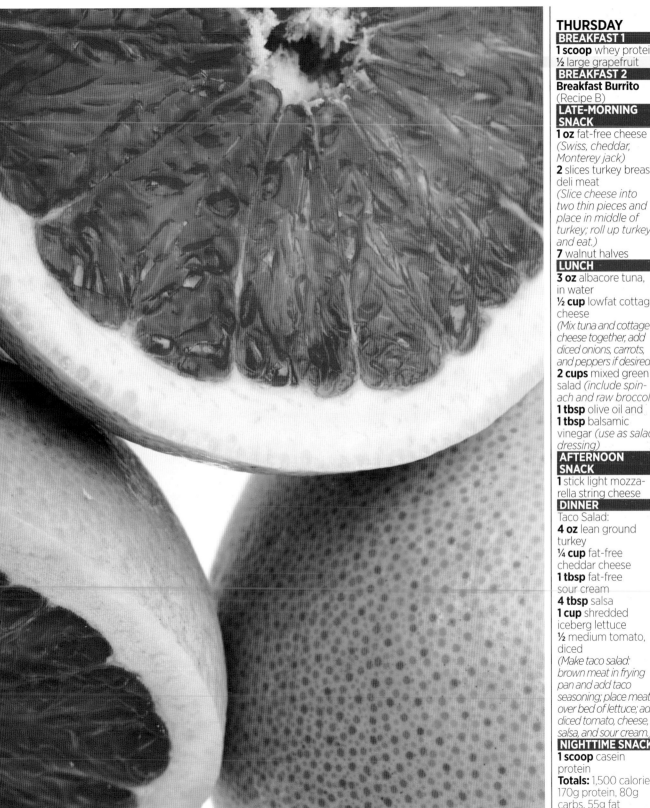

THURSDAY

BREAKFAST 1
1 scoop whey protein
½ large grapefruit

BREAKFAST 2
Breakfast Burrito
(Recipe B)

LATE-MORNING SNACK
1 oz fat-free cheese
(Swiss, cheddar, Monterey jack)
2 slices turkey breast deli meat
(Slice cheese into two thin pieces and place in middle of turkey; roll up turkey and eat.)
7 walnut halves

LUNCH
3 oz albacore tuna, in water
½ cup lowfat cottage cheese
(Mix tuna and cottage cheese together, add diced onions, carrots, and peppers if desired.)
2 cups mixed green salad *(include spinach and raw broccoli)*
1 tbsp olive oil and
1 tbsp balsamic vinegar *(use as salad dressing)*

AFTERNOON SNACK
1 stick light mozzarella string cheese

DINNER
Taco Salad:
4 oz lean ground turkey
¼ cup fat-free cheddar cheese
1 tbsp fat-free sour cream
4 tbsp salsa
1 cup shredded iceberg lettuce
½ medium tomato, diced
(Make taco salad: brown meat in frying pan and add taco seasoning; place meat over bed of lettuce; add diced tomato, cheese, salsa, and sour cream.)

NIGHTTIME SNACK
1 scoop casein protein

Totals: 1,500 calories, 170g protein, 80g carbs, 55g fat

FRIDAY

BREAKFAST 1
1 scoop whey protein
½ large grapefruit

BREAKFAST 2
½ cup low-fat milk
½ cup Kashi Go Lean cereal
2 large whole eggs *(scrambled, fried, or hard-boiled)*

LATE-MORNING SNACK
¼ cup boiled soybeans (aka edamame)
1 stick light mozzarella string cheese

LUNCH
¾ cup low-fat cottage cheese *(Mix in any desired vegetables.)*

MIDDAY SNACK
4 oz shrimp
1 tbsp seafood cocktail sauce

DINNER
Chili Con Carne *(Recipe C)*
2 cups mixed green salad *(include spinach and raw broccoli)*
1 tbsp olive oil and **1 tbsp** balsamic vinegar *(use as salad dressing)*

NIGHTTIME SNACK
1 scoop casein protein
2 medium celery stalks
1 tbsp peanut butter *(Spread peanut butter into grooves of celery.)*
Totals: 1,600 calories, 170g protein, 75g carbs, 65g fat

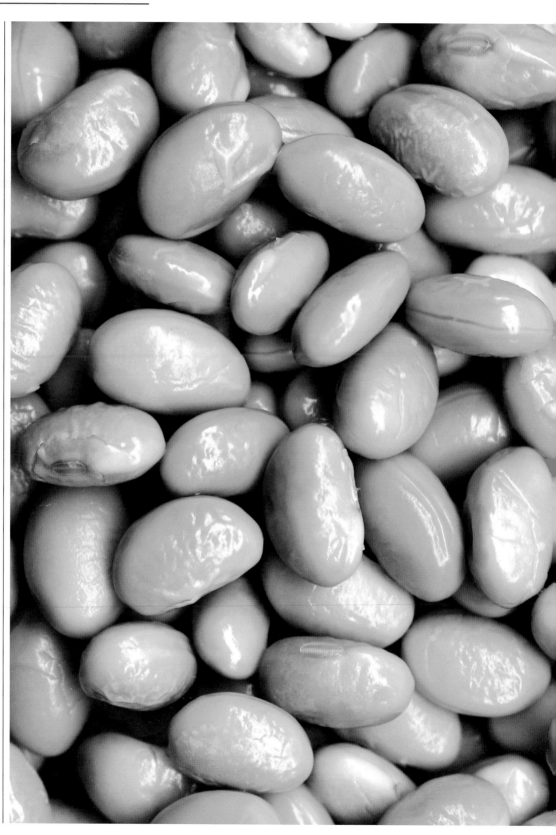

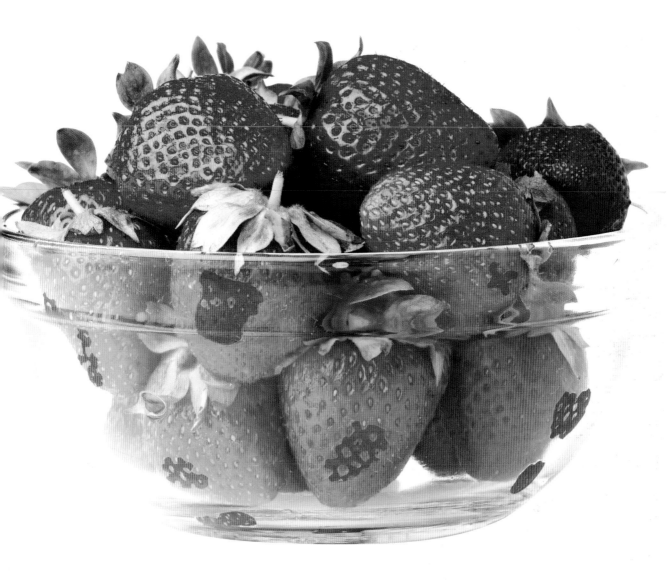

SATURDAY

BREAKFAST 1
1 scoop whey protein
1 large grapefruit

BREAKFAST 2
Omelet (Recipe D)
**1 whole-wheat
English muffin
1 tbsp peanut butter

LATE-MORNING SNACK
1 stick light mozzarella string cheese
1 medium celery stalks
1 tbsp peanut butter
(Spread peanut butter into grooves of celery.)

LUNCH
3 oz albacore tuna, in water
1 tbsp light mayonnaise
3 whole-wheat crackers
(Add any desired vegetables to tuna salad and eat with crackers.)

MIDDAY SNACK
½ cup reduced-fat Greek yogurt
7 walnut halves
(Mix walnuts in yogurt.)

DINNER
6 oz salmon

1 cup cooked cauliflower
2 cups mixed green salad *(include spinach and raw broccoli)*
1 tbsp olive oil and
1 tbsp balsamic vinegar *(use as salad dressing)*

NIGHTTIME SNACK
¾ cup low-fat cottage cheese
Totals: 1,635 calories, 150g protein, 75g carbs, 85g fat

SUNDAY (High-carb "cheat" day)

BREAKFAST 1
1 scoop whey protein
1 large grapefruit

BREAKFAST 2
Breakfast Pizza (Recipe E)
4 oz (½ cup) orange juice

LATE-MORNING SNACK
8 oz nonfat fruit yogurt

LUNCH
3 oz albacore tuna, in water
1 tbsp fat-free mayonnaise

1 large (6.5") pita bread (white)
(Mix mayo in tuna to make tuna salad, and add any veggies you desire. Scoop tuna salad into pita bread.)
1 cup sliced strawberries
4 tbsp fat-free Reddi-Wip

MIDDAY SNACK
1½ cups Kashi Go Lean cereal
1 cup low-fat milk

DINNER
4 oz chicken breast
1 large sweet potato

2 tbsp fat-free sour cream
(Top potato with sour cream.)
2 cups mixed green salad *(include spinach and raw broccoli)*
1 tbsp olive oil and
1 tbsp balsamic vinegar *(use as salad dressing)*

NIGHTTIME SNACK
1 scoop casein protein
1 cup cooked oatmeal
Totals: 2,260 calories, 190g protein, 300g carbs, 40g fat

THE 15 BEST FAT-BURNING FOODS

1) WALNUTS
All nuts do contain some amount of the omega-3 fat alpha-linolenic acid, but most contain only trace amounts. The real fat hero in most nuts is monounsaturated fats, such as omega-3s. Walnuts are actually a rich source of this healthy fat. One ounce provides almost 3g of alpha-linolenic acid.

2) GINGER
Used for centuries to help relieve digestive upset/disturbances, ginger can also help reduce inflammation, boost blood flow to muscles, and aid muscle recovery. It has also has been shown to boost calorie burn when eaten.

3) OATMEAL
This very-slow-digesting carb keeps blood sugar and insulin levels low, so fat burning can stay high. In fact, research has shown that athletes who consume slow-digesting carbs in the morning burn more fat throughout the entire day and during workouts than those consuming fast-digesting carbs.

4) AVOCADO
The monounsaturated fats found in avocados are burned readily for fuel during exercise and actually encourage fat burning. Avocados also contain a very interesting carb called mannoheptulose, a sugar that actually blunts insulin release and enhances calcium absorption, both of which are critical for encouraging fat loss.

STUDY IT
Research shows that endurance athletes who maintain a low-carb diet for several weeks perform just as well on low carbs as they did on high carbs, but only after a few weeks of restricting carbs.

5) SALMON
This fish is one of the richest sources of the omega-3 essential fats EPA and DHA. Unlike flaxseeds, which provide a type of omega-3 that has to be converted into EPA and DHA, salmon provides your body a direct supply of them with no conversion required. This way you know you're getting a direct supply of the fats that turn on fat burning and block fat storage.

6) SOYBEANS (EDAMAME)
Soybeans are the direct origin of so protein, which has been shown to build muscle as efficiently as other forms of protein like whey and beef. Soy has also bee shown to aid fat loss, possibly by decreasing appetite and calorie intake.

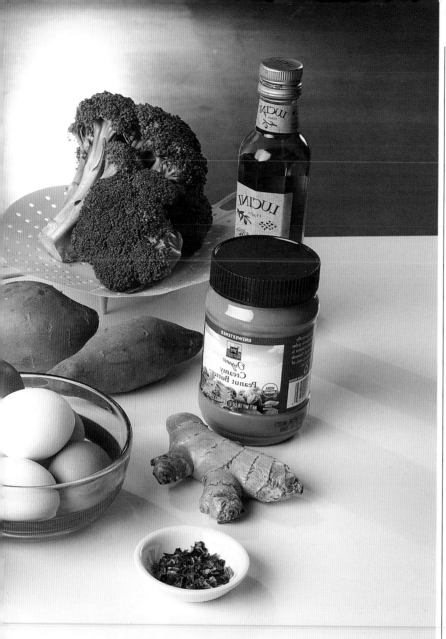

9) GRAPEFRUIT

A study from the Scripps Clinic (San Diego, CA) reported that subjects eating half of a grapefruit or drinking 8 oz of grapefruit juice three times a day while maintaining their normal diet lost an average of 4 pounds over 12 weeks—and some lost more than 10 pounds without even dieting! Results were likely due to grapefruit's ability to reduce insulin levels, and to a chemical in grapefruit known as naringin, which prevents fat from being stored in the body.

10) HONEY

Yes, it's a sugar, but it's fairly low on the glycemic index. Keeping insulin levels low and steady is critical for maintaining a fat-burning environment in your body. Honey is also a rich source of nitric oxide (NO) metabolites; ultimately, that means it actually encourages fat release from the body's fat cells.

11) PEANUT BUTTER

Another source of helpful mono-unsaturated fat that can actually aid fat loss. What's funny is that many food manufacturers make low-fat peanut butters! Of course, they replace these healthy mono-unsaturated fats with carbs, namely sugar. Avoid these and stick with natural peanut butters that don't add the types of fat you surely want to avoid—trans fats.

12) EGGS

Yes, we listed eggs in the muscle-building foods section later in this chapter. So how can it also be a fat-burning food? Research supports the notion that those who start their day with eggs not only eat fewer calories throughout the day, but also lose significantly more body fat.

13) CHILI PEPPER FLAKES

Hot peppers contain the active ingredient capsaicin, a chemical that can enhance calorie burning at rest as well as reduce hunger and food intake. The boost in calorie burn is particularly enhanced when capsaicin is used with caffeine.

14) BROCCOLI

This fibrous carb doesn't provide many net carbs or calories, but it can make you feel full—one reason why it's a great food for getting lean. Broccoli also contains phytochemicals that can help enhance fat loss.

15) OLIVE OIL

Like avocados, olive oil is a great source of monounsaturated fats. Not only do they lower levels of the "bad" type of cholesterol and improve cardiovascular health, but they're also more likely to be burned as fuel, which means they're less likely to be sticking around your midsection.

7) WATER

This just may be your best ally in fighting body fat. Studies have shown that drinking 2 cups of cold water can boost metabolic rate by 30%. It has been estimated that drinking about 2 cups of cold water before breakfast, lunch, and dinner every day for a year can burn 17,400 extra calories, which translates into a little more than 5 pounds of body fat!

8) FLAXSEEDS

They contain the essential omega-3 fatty acid alpha linolenic acid. These omega-3 fats have been found to turn on genes that stimulate fat burning and turn off genes that increase fat storage.

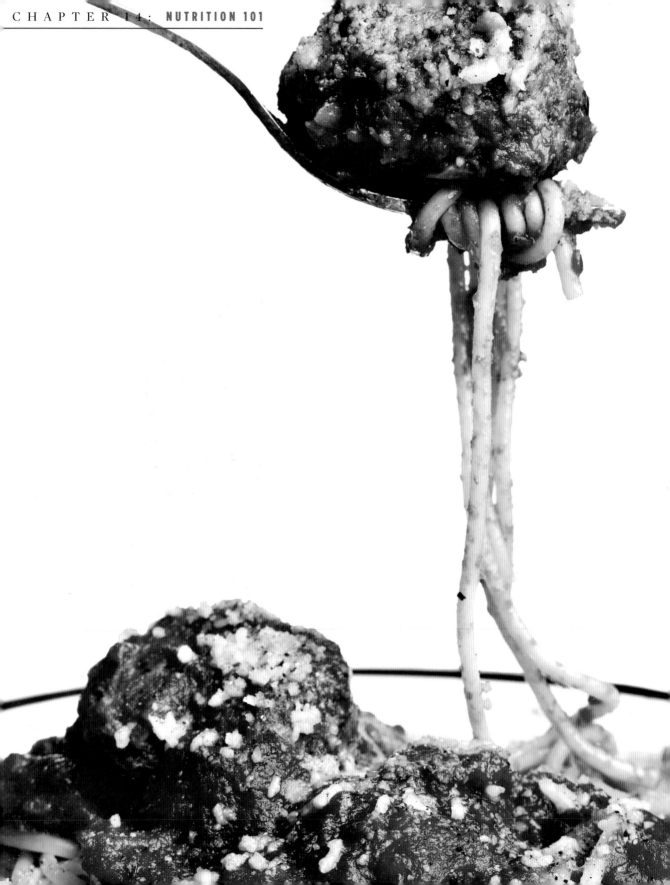

GOAL: BUILD LEAN MUSCLE ONE-WEEK MEAL PLAN

The following plan is designed for a woman weighing 140 pounds. When trying to gain lean muscle during a rigorous exercise program, a good rule of thumb is to shoot for an intake of about 13–15 calories per pound of body weight. So for a 110-pound woman, total daily calories would be between 1,430 to 1,650; for a 150-pound woman, about 1,950 to 2,250.

A FRITTATA

large whole eggs
arge egg white
cup low-fat cottage cheese
cup chopped broccoli
medium onion (chopped)
frying pan on medium heat,
ook onions for about five min-
es with fat-free cooking spray;
ld broccoli and cook for about
e minutes; in a large bowl, mix
ggs and cottage cheese and
ld to pan, and then lift and ro-
te pan so that eggs are evenly
stributed; as eggs set around
e edges, lift to allow uncooked
ortions to flow underneath.
Irn heat to low, cover the
an and cook until top is set.
vert onto a plate.

B STIR-FRY

4 oz shrimp
1 large whole egg
½ cup cooked medium-grain
brown rice
1 cup mixed frozen veggies
Spray pan with nonfat cooking
spray, then cook shrimp over
medium heat, add boiled rice
and vegetables, add scrambled
egg and soy sauce if desired
and cook for about 5 to 10 minutes, stirring frequently.

C SPAGHETTI AND MEATBALLS

4 oz lean ground turkey
1 cup cooked spaghetti squash
¼ cup fat-free ricotta
Mix desired spices with ground
turkey and roll into balls; add
desired spices to sauce and cook
meatballs in sauce until done.
Cook spaghetti squash in a shal-
low baking pan with ½ inch of
water in pan at 350 degrees in
oven until tender. Scrape out spaghetti squash with fork to make
spaghetti strings. Top spaghetti
squash with meatballs and sauce,

D BREAKFAST SANDWICH

1 large whole egg
1 slice reduced-fat
American cheese
2 slices low-fat deli ham
1 whole-wheat English muffin
Toast muffin; fry ham in pan
and place on one half of muffin;
fry egg in pan using nonstick
cooking spray and place on ham;
top egg with cheese and cover
with other muffin half to make
breakfast sandwich.

MONDAY

BREAKFAST 1
1 scoop whey protein
½ small/medium cantaloupe

BREAKFAST 2
(30–60 minutes after B1)
2 large whole eggs
2 slices low-fat deli ham
¼ cup fat-free cheddar cheese
(Make ham and cheese omelet.)
1 cup cooked oatmeal

LATE-MORNING SNACK
4 oz reduced-fat Greek yogurt
½ cup blueberries
(Mix blueberries in yogurt.)

LUNCH
4 oz lean ground beef
1 whole-wheat hamburger bun
2 cups mixed green salad *(include spinach)*
1 tbsp olive oil and
1 tbsp balsamic vinegar *(use as salad dressing)*

MIDDAY SNACK
3 oz can chicken breast *(such as Swanson)*
1 tbsp light mayonnaise
5 whole-wheat crackers
(Mix mayo in chicken; eat on crackers.)

DINNER
6 oz chicken breast
1 cup chopped broccoli
2 cups mixed green salad *(include spinach)*
1 tbsp olive oil and
1 tbsp balsamic vinegar *(use as salad dressing)*

NIGHTTIME SNACK
¾ cup cottage cheese
2 tbsp salsa
(Mix salsa in cottage cheese.)
Totals: 1,835 calories, 185g protein, 135g carbs, 65g fat

TUESDAY

BREAKFAST 1
1 scoop whey protein
1 large orange

BREAKFAST 2
2 large whole eggs
2 large egg whites
(Make scrambled eggs.)
1 whole-grain waffle *(such as Van's)*
1 tbsp maple syrup

LATE-MORNING SNACK
1 scoop whey protein
½ cup wheat germ
(Mix wheat germ in whey shake.)

LUNCH
4 oz turkey deli meat
1 tbsp light mayonnaise
2 slices Ezekiel 4:9 bread
(Combine to make turkey sandwich.)

MIDDAY SNACK
½ cup low-fat cottage cheese
¼ cup sliced pineapple
(Mix pineapple in cottage cheese.)

DINNER
6 oz tilapia
1 cup broccoli
2 cups mixed green salad *(include spinach)*
1 tbsp olive oil and
1 tbsp balsamic vinegar *(use as salad dressing)*

NIGHTTIME SNACK
1 scoop casein protein
7 walnut halves
1 tbsp peanut butter
(Dip walnuts in peanut butter.)
Totals: 1,870 calories, 190g protein, 145g carbs, 60g fat

WEDNESDAY

BREAKFAST 1
1 scoop whey protein
1 small apple

BREAKFAST 2
Frittata (Recipe A)
1 cup cooked oatmeal

LATE-MORNING SNACK
½ cup reduced-fat Greek yogurt
½ cup sliced strawberries

LUNCH
Stir-fry (Recipe B)

MIDDAY SNACK
½ cup low-fat cottage cheese
½ cup canned Mandarin oranges

DINNER
6 oz top sirloin steak
20 asparagus spears
2 cups mixed green salad *(include spinach)*
1 tbsp olive oil and
1 tbsp balsamic vinegar *(use as salad dressing)*

NIGHTTIME SNACK
1 cup reduced-fat Greek yogurt
1 tsp honey
2 tbsp roasted flaxseeds
(Mix honey and flaxseeds in yogurt.)

Totals: 1,900 calories, 180g protein, 160g carbs, 55g fat

THURSDAY

BREAKFAST 1
1 scoop whey protein
½ medium cantaloupe

BREAKFAST 2
½ cup low-fat milk
½ cup Kashi Go Lean cereal
½ scoop whey protein

LATE-MORNING SNACK
2 cups mixed green salad *(include spinach)*
2 large whole eggs, hard-boiled and sliced
¼ cup dry oatmeal
1 tbsp olive oil and
1 tbsp balsamic vinegar *(use as salad dressing)*
(Make salad by adding all ingredients together.)

LUNCH
5 oz packet sea-soned tuna filets
(such as StarKist)
½ cup cooked quinoa
1 cup mixed frozen veggies

MIDDAY SNACK
10" whole-wheat pita *(such as Missio. Foods)*
¼ cup reduced-fat cheddar cheese shredded
(Add cheese to one side of tortilla, fold in half, and cook on medium heat in frying pan until cheese is melted.)

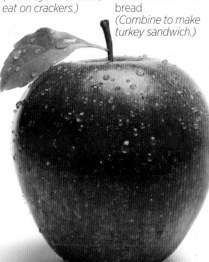

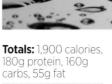

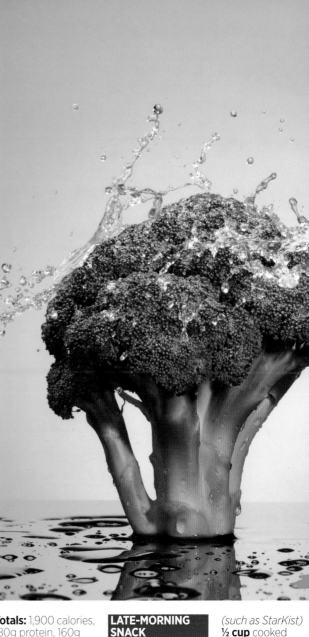

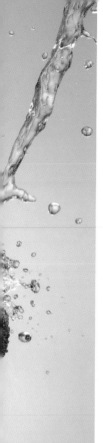

FRIDAY

BREAKFAST 1
1 scoop whey protein
1 small apple

BREAKFAST 2
¾ cup cottage cheese
½ cup canned Mandarin oranges
2 medium stalks celery
1 tbsp peanut butter
(Fill celery grooves with peanut butter.)

LATE-MORNING SNACK
1 scoop whey protein
½ cup wheat germ
(Mix whey and wheat germ together.)

LUNCH
4 oz turkey breast deli meat
1 slice reduced-fat American cheese
1 tbsp light mayonnaise
10" whole-wheat pita

MIDDAY SNACK
2 oz fat-free cheese
5 whole-wheat crackers

DINNER
6 oz tilapia
2 cups mixed green salad *(include spinach)*
1 tbsp olive oil and
1 tbsp balsamic vinegar *(use as salad dressing)*

NIGHTTIME SNACK
1 scoop casein protein
7 walnut halves
Totals: 1,915 calories, 195g protein, 145g carbs, 65g fat

SATURDAY

BREAKFAST 1
1 scoop whey protein
1 large orange

BREAKFAST 2
2 large whole eggs
2 large egg whites
¼ cup reduced-fat cheddar cheese, shredded
(Combine to make cheese omelet.)
1 whole-wheat English muffin
1 tbsp peanut butter
(Spread peanut butter on toasted muffin.)

LATE-MORNING SNACK
½ cup boiled soybeans
1 cup chicken noodle soup

LUNCH
3 oz albacore tuna, in water
2 cups mixed green salad *(include spinach)*
1 cup canned beets

1 oz fat-free feta cheese
1 tbsp olive oil and
1 tbsp balsamic vinegar *(use as salad dressing)*
½ large whole-wheat pita bread, sliced into wedges
(Add ingredients to salad and eat with pita bread.)

MIDDAY SNACK
1 cup reduced-fat

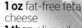

Greek yogurt
1 tbsp honey

DINNER
Spaghetti and Meatballs (Recipe C)

NIGHTTIME SNACK
¾ cup cottage cheese
Totals: 2,000 calories, 180g protein, 170g carbs, 70g fat

SUNDAY *(High-carb "cheat" day)*

BREAKFAST 1
1 scoop whey protein
½ medium cantaloupe

BREAKFAST 2
Breakfast Sandwich (Recipe D)

LATE-MORNING SNACK
½ cup reduced-fat Greek yogurt
½ cup blueberries

LUNCH
4 oz turkey deli meat
2 slices Ezekiel 4:9 bread

2 cups mixed green salad *(include spinach)*
1 tbsp olive oil and
1 tbsp balsamic vinegar *(use as salad dressing)*

MIDDAY SNACK
½ 10" whole-wheat pita *(Mission Foods)*
¼ cup fat-free cheddar
(Make cheese quesadilla.)

DINNER (CHEAT MEAL)
3 slices pepperoni pizza
12-oz Budweiser
1 cup ice cream

NIGHTTIME SNACK
½ cup low-fat cottage cheese
2 tbsp salsa
Totals: 2,500 calories, 160g protein, 255g carbs, 75g fat

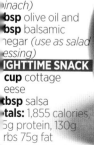

DINNER
oz salmon
cups mixed green salad *(include spinach)*
bsp olive oil and
bsp balsamic vinegar *(use as salad dressing)*

NIGHTTIME SNACK
cup cottage cheese
tbsp salsa
tals: 1,855 calories, 5g protein, 130g rbs 75g fat

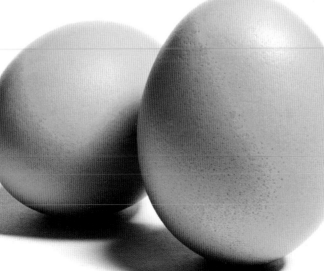

THE 15 BEST LEAN-MUSCLE-BUILDING FOODS

1) BEEF (FROM GRASS-FED CATTLE)
Beef is important for building lean muscle due to its protein content, cholesterol, zinc, B vitamins, and iron content. Beef from grass-fed cattle has much higher levels of conjugated linoleic acid (CLA) than conventionally raised cattle beef, which gives you a boost in shedding body fat and building lean muscle.

2) BEETS
A good source of betaine, also known as trimethylglycine, this nutrient not only enhances liver and joint repair, but also has been shown in clinical research to increase muscle strength and power. Beets also provide an nitric oxide boost which can enhance energy and aid recovery.

3) BROWN RICE
A slow-digesting whole grain that provides you longer-lasting energy throughout the day, and during workouts. Brown rice also can help boost your growth hormone (GH) levels, which are critical for encouraging lean muscle growth, fat loss, and strength gains.

4) ORANGES
Another good fruit that can actually help to boost muscle growth, strength, and endurance, especially when eaten before workouts.

5) CANTALOUPE
Due to it's relatively low fructose content, this melon is one of the few fruits that is actually a fast-digesting carb. That makes it a good carb to have first thing in the morning after a long night of fasting, or after a tough workout, when your muscles' glycogen fuel stores are depleted.

6) COTTAGE CHEESE (ORGANIC)
Rich in casein protein, cottage cheese is a great go-to protein source, especially before bed. Casein protein is the slowest-digesting protein you can eat, meaning it prevents your muscles from being used as an energy source while you fast during the night.

7) EGGS
Eggs are known as the perfect protein, but their ability to boost lean muscle and strength gains isn't due to just the protein alone. They get a lot of help from the yolks, where the cholesterol is found. If you're worried about your cholesterol shooting up from eating the yolks, cholesterol from eggs has been shown to actually decrease the amount of LDL (bad) cholesterol particles associated with atherosclerosis (hardened arteries).

8) MILK (ORGANIC)
Contains both whey and casein and is rich in the amino acid glutamine. Organic milk has about 70% more omega-3 fatty acids than conventional milk.

9) QUINOA
A complete protein in addition to being a slow-digesting carb, quinoa has been linked with an increase in insulin-like growth factor-1 (IGF-1) levels, an important factor associated with lean muscle and strength gains.

10) WONKA PIXY STIX
These contain dextrose, meaning this carb doesn't even need to be digested—it literally goes straight into your bloodstream, getting those carbs straight to your muscles for the fastest recovery possible after workouts.

11) SPINACH
A good source of glutamine, the amino acid that is important for lean muscle growth. In addition to glutamine spinach can increase muscle strength and endurance.

12) APPLES
The specific polyphenols in apples help to increase muscle strength and prevent muscle fatigue, allowing you to train harder for longer. Other research also shows that these polyphenols can increase fat burning as well. That's why it's a good idea to make apples a pre-workout carb source.

13) GREEK YOGURT
Like plain yogurt, Greek yogurt starts from the same source: milk. Greek yogurt, however, has more protein (a whopping 20g per cup) and fewer carbs (9g per cup) than regular yogurt (16g protein, 16g carbs per cup). It's also a good source of casein protein.

14) EZEKIEL 4:9 BREAD
Ezekiel bread is made from organic sprouted whole grains. Because it contains grains and legumes, the bread is a complete protein, which means it contains all nine of the amino acids your body can't produce on its own—the ones needed for lean muscle growth.

15) WHEAT GERM
Rich in zinc, iron, selenium, potassium, and B vitamins; high in fiber and protein, with a good amount of branched-chain amino acids (BCAAs), arginine, and glutamine. This makes wheat germ a great source of slow-digesting carbohydrates and a quality protein that's a perfect food before workouts.

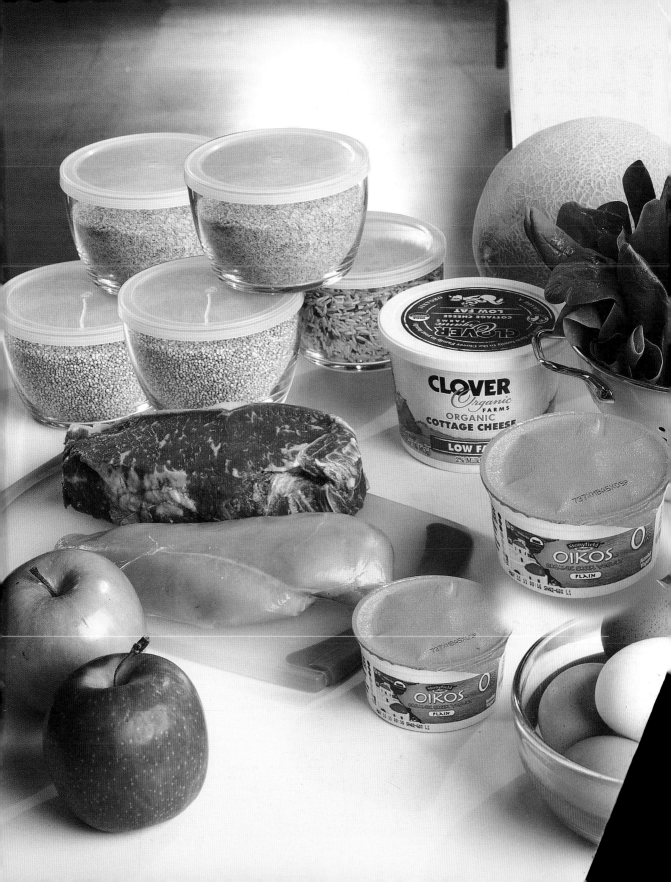